Psychology Revivals

Nursing Psychological Patients

Originally published in 1931, *Nursing Psychological Patients* was 'a book written by a nurse for the purpose of increasing the interest of members of the nursing profession in psychological diseases, by pointing out that they require the nurses' serious attention and offer an important field for professional skill. The opening chapters summarize former opinions and earlier methods of treating this group of human sufferings, and trace the subsequent growth of knowledge and the development of modern forms of treatment. Later chapters describe the more familiar neurotic troubles, their symptoms and the difficulties they present to the nurse, and attempt, by increasing her understanding, to render her more efficient in meeting wisely the problems which she encounters.' Today it can be read in its historical context.

This book is a re-issue originally published in 1931. The language used is a reflection of its era and no offence is meant by the Publishers to any reader by this re-publication.

Nursing Psychological Patients

Mary Chadwick

Routledge
Taylor & Francis Group
LONDON AND NEW YORK

First published in 1931
by George Allen & Unwin Ltd

This edition first published in 2025 by Routledge
4 Park Square, Milton Park, Abingdon, Oxon, OX14 4RN

and by Routledge
605 Third Avenue, New York, NY 10017

Routledge is an imprint of the Taylor & Francis Group, an informa business

Publisher's Note
The publisher has gone to great lengths to ensure the quality of this reprint but points out that some imperfections in the original copies may be apparent.

Disclaimer
The publisher has made every effort to trace copyright holders and welcomes correspondence from those they have been unable to contact.

A Library of Congress record exists under LCCN: 33006305

ISBN: 978-1-041-04750-6 (hbk)
ISBN: 978-1-003-62974-0 (ebk)
ISBN: 978-1-041-04763-6 (pbk)

Book DOI 10.4324/9781003629740

NURSING PSYCHOLOGICAL PATIENTS

by

MARY CHADWICK, S.R.N.

Foreword by

DAVID FORSYTH, M.D., D.SC., F.R.C.P.

Senior Physician, Charing Cross Hospital; Consulting Physician, Evelina Hospital; Late Senior Physician, Psychological Clinic, Ministry of Pensions (London)

LONDON

GEORGE ALLEN & UNWIN LTD

MUSEUM STREET

FIRST PUBLISHED IN 1931

PRINTED IN GREAT BRITAIN BY
UNWIN BROTHERS LTD., WOKING

DEDICATED TO

THE NURSING STAFF OF THE

UNIVERSITY COLLEGE HOSPITAL, LONDON

WHERE THESE LECTURES WERE FIRST GIVEN IN

APRIL AND MAY, 1928

AND TO ALL OTHERS INTERESTED IN

THIS IMPORTANT SUBJECT

PREFACE

In reading present-day textbooks upon Nursing, one is struck by the lack of up-to-date information concerning that large section of patients needing the Nurse's care who are suffering from some form of Psychological Trouble. The last twenty-five years or more of medical research have added greatly to the knowledge which is available for their benefit; moreover, many new ways of curing and alleviating these ailments have been introduced. Still, as yet, no one has seen fit to equip the Nurse with a handbook that may help her to care for these sick folk adequately and intelligently.

A few years back an attempt was made to give a summary of the contribution which applied psychology, and especially *psycho-analysis*, has bestowed upon medical science for the treatment and understanding of those who are suffering from abnormal psychogenic conditions in a small volume entitled *Psychology for Nurses*; but whereas this endeavoured to give the Nurse some understanding as to the present state of her patient and the usual causes of the symptoms which arise, no special nursing methods are described, nor are the principles underlying their nursing indicated.

The nursing of those troubled with Psychological Disorders is far more complicated and arduous than that of other cases which may be classified under the heading of Medical or Surgical Nursing, and yet it is seldom indeed that these illnesses are not complicated by some symptoms of neurotic origin, which are often passed over as of little importance or may even be unrecognised, although they will frequently be responsible for delay in expected convalescence or the recovery of complete health.

The object of this book is to explain the state of affairs in the most general forms of psychological disorders in such a way that the Nurse, by understanding what lies behind the manifest symptoms of the trouble, may more easily and adequately help her patients, as well as find the work less worrying and tedious to herself. It is commonly stated by the generality of Nurses that they would rather nurse a surgical case of great severity than one of nervous origin, although they are usually unable to give any reason why this should be so. The difficulty, however, usually lies in this fact, that when nursing the former they feel they have a better understanding of the course of the illness, and also because their part of the work has been more definitely described to them. Not so with the nursing of the Nervous Patient. Here the Nurse does *not* understand the course of the illness; she has no clear instructions to carry out, and it frequently happens that a method of treatment which has been successful in the case of one patient supposed to be suffering from the same trouble is useless in another.

MARY CHADWICK

48, Tavistock Square
London, W.C.1

FOREWORD

This new book of Miss Mary Chadwick's is one that I can warmly recommend. It comes first in the field in bringing the signal advances in recent medical psychology under the special notice of the nursing profession. On internal evidence it proves that the author has both read widely and kept herself up to date in a subject which is still growing fast. Her earlier contributions to psychology, some of them original, show that her studies have been by no means theoretical only, and the practical utility of this book is apparent throughout.

I wish I could dissent from Miss Chadwick's stricture that most nurses do not understand neurotic cases; but I cannot. Whether in hospital or nursing-home it is rare in my experience to meet with a nurse who has any appreciation of the problems involved in cases of this kind. And yet an informed nurse can be as helpful to a doctor in a "nerve case" as in any medical or surgical case. It is in the knowledge of this that I hopefully anticipate that the author's purpose will be successful, and that this book will foster in very many of its readers an intelligent and sympathetic interest in a class of patients which has hitherto been undeservedly disparaged. Its further aim seems to me to be no less commendable—to educate public opinion by the agency of an educated nursing opinion. In this way it should give an increased velocity to that slow process of disabusing the lay mind of its present queer notions about mental illness.

DAVID FORSYTH

May 1931

CONTENTS

NAMES, COUNTRIES, AND METHODS

ASSOCIATED WITH THE TREATMENT OF PSYCHOLOGICAL DISORDERS

Name	Country or Centre	Method
Galen. A.D. 130–200	Greece	Various
Culpeper. b. 1653	England	Various
Mesmer. 1734–1815	Vienna and Paris	Mesmerism
John Elliotson. 1791–1868	England	Hypnotism
James Esdaile. 1808–1859	England	Hypnotism
James Braid. 1795–1860	England	Hypnotism
Dr. A. A. Liébeault. b. 1823	France	Hypnotism with Suggestion
Bernheim	France	Hypnotism with Suggestion
Charcot. 1825–1893	France	Hypnotism with Suggestion
Janet	France	Hypnotism with Suggestion
Josef Breuer	Vienna	Cathartic Treatment
Sigmund Freud. b. 1856	Vienna	Psycho-analysis
Alfred Adler	Vienna	Individual Psychology
C. G. Jung	Zürich	Analytical Psychology
W. Erb	Germany	Electro-therapy
J. Babinski	Paris and London	Electro-therapy
G. W. Crile. b. 1864	America	Anocio-association
S. Weir-Mitchell. 1830–1914	America	Rest-cures
Emile Coué	France	Auto-suggestion

SYNOPSIS OF CONTENTS

CHAPTER I

CHAPTER II

CHAPTER III

CHAPTER IV

CHAPTER V

CHAPTER VI

PSYCHOLOGICAL DISORDERS COMMON AMONG MEN AND BOYS—(*continued*)

ALCOHOLISM AND DRUG ADDICTION

Underlying idea to supply an emotional deficiency. Roots of this craving. Can a healthier substitute or compensation be found?

WAR SHOCK

Usually not the first neurotic manifestation in the life of the patient.

Handicap to recovery of the secondary gain of illness. How best to nurse these patients.

Need for abreaction of repressed emotions and provision of outlets for fundamental impulses.

NURSING PSYCHOLOGICAL PATIENTS

NURSING PSYCHOLOGICAL PATIENTS

CHAPTER I

INTRODUCTORY

History of Former Treatment of Psychological Disorders

We are inclined to believe that the group of human sickness to which the name Psycho-neuroses has been given is in some way a modern invention, that it is a result of over-civilisation and the consequence of present-day restlessness, or the evils of *speeding-up*. Yet, should we examine medical records of bygone days, we find that this is by no means the case. The troubles will, it is true, be known to the modern practitioner by different names; recent research has ascribed a different origin to their chief symptoms, and the doctor, if thoroughly up to date, prescribes a different method of treating his patient. Should he be as fond of adhering to old forms of therapy as were his professional ancestors, he may even now, however, curiously enough, order remedies which bear a strange resemblance to those that were the outcome of early beliefs.

Although actual methods have undergone considerable changes during the centuries that have elapsed since we first find definite mention of these diseases in medical treatises, they remain constant in this one respect, that the recognised remedies always bear a direct relation to the accepted theories of the cause of the trouble which were then prevalent. For instance, savage races have always regarded sick persons with abhorrence or religious awe, except those whose illness was clearly the outcome of wounds inflicted by an enemy or a wild beast, and left them to be dealt with by the medicine-man, who originally was half priest, half doctor. Modern eugenists try to persuade us that the primitive instinct to slay the physically unfit was due to an instinctive wish to keep the health of the tribe as untainted as possible; but recent psychological research exposes a somewhat different motive to this primitive attitude to disease that had no external cause, and especially to those which we now regard as nervous or mental.

It would now seem that these stimulated intense *fear*, arising from a sense of *guilt*, never far distant from the primitive mind in relation to anything the cause of which was unknown, both in those who looked on as well as in the patients themselves. This sense of guilt immediately ascribed the troubles to direct intervention of an angry deity, as retribution for wrong-doing on the part of the patient or his family. This belief, therefore, greatly influenced the treatment of these sufferers in many ways, since the nervous diseases, more than any others, seemed to portray divine vengeance. Whenever it was possible they were treated as though the complaint were physical, and the medicine-man attempted to withdraw the disease in some way, occasionally by sucking the evil out, as we might now foment an abscess to extract pus. His success to accomplish this he would prove to the populace by showing a crystal which he had secreted in his mouth before he commenced operations, or he used what we should now call some form of suggestion. But when such methods failed, guilt and fear became intolerant, and he insisted that patients should be banished to prevent contamination of the tribe. In this way they were often shunned rather than helped in those far-off days, although they may not have been actively molested as were the insane, who might also prove a menace to the bodily welfare of the community.

Among these abnormal conditions which seem to have been prevalent among ancient peoples we may group those known to-day as melancholia, acute depression; hysterical attacks, or those of an epileptoid nature; obsessional neuroses, early forms of dementia præcox and mania; those, in truth, which we now often regard as *borderline cases.* It is a curious fact that many of the medicine-men themselves suffered from slight manifestations of these same diseases, in which case the epileptiform attack would be taken as evidence of miraculous power and the indisputable presence of the god within his priest. Yet, when these same symptoms appeared among the common people, they were assumed to be the sign of the anger of the deity on account of some misdeed of the patient or his parents, in which case the illness represented punishment or expiation for the sin, so that it would then be interference with the divine power to seek a remedy for the affliction.

It is interesting to note that to this day we find a strong sense of guilt as well as fear of divine retribution in those who suffer from these same maladies, although in many cases they know of no cause which justifies their belief. The origin remains buried in their unconscious mind, and only appears after investigation has been made by experts through special methods. The realisation of guiltiness, however, has to a great measure the same effect as in the past, in one respect. It still hinders the possibility of the cure, although at present this reluctance comes mainly from the side of the patient, who will often feel that the affliction of God should be borne with patience, and that to seek relief might show lack of faith in His actions being for the best. Although this idea may not be so clearly expressed now as in the past, we find it often prevents a patient or his relatives following up information that treatment for the cure or alleviation of the troubles is available. Or, should the patient be a child, the parents will frequently say: "What have I done to be afflicted with such a child?" or, "What can this child have done to have to suffer like this?" which shows that a hypothetical connection between illness, guilt, and sin is by no means only a mental curiosity existing among savages, but a phenomenon of the *primitive mind,* which survives to some extent in us all, and tends to come to the surface respecting these abnormal states, which we call *neuroses* or *psycho-neuroses.*

Several abnormal psychological conditions were recognised and distinguished one from another during the dawn of modern medicine by the first Greek physicians, and it is interesting to compare the observations left to us in early medical works with the symptoms presented by similar conditions found in our patients to-day. Their observation and description of the clinical picture presented by their patients makes it quite possible to recognise distinct types of neurotic disorder we still find among those we are called upon to nurse to-day; but the complaints are usually given a different name, and the causes to which the symptoms were then ascribed strike us now as highly fanciful. Remedies which were prescribed were the logical sequence of their belief in the accuracy of the diagnosed cause, but often seem to us as too childish for credence, while many other types of similar troubles must have been left entirely unalleviated or even untreated.

Greek Theories. Galen. A.D. 130–200

The first psycho-neurosis to be accorded an honourable place in the history of medicine was that of *Hysteria,* so called from the Greek word for the womb, since the typical condition of emotional instability, which was then, as now, associated with this trouble, was supposed to be caused by the wandering of this organ about the interior of the body. In those days it was naturally for this reason regarded as a complaint occurring only in women, which calls to mind the hostility with which medical men in the past, who were unwilling to accept new ideas, opposed any suggestions that similar symptoms might also be found in males. With this theory in view—the vagaries of the uterus—treatment consisted of attempts to keep this errant organ in place. Evil-smelling drugs were administered to frighten it into good behaviour or to prevent the patient finding her affliction too interesting may be, or too convenient, as an escape from other difficult situations. But this latter interpretation was not taken into direct consideration by the ancient Greek physicians as its motive, although the unpleasant remedy most probably had the more beneficial effect through the influence of this psychological channel than that which was formerly stated, i.e. to frighten the womb into docile passivity. (See note at the end of this chapter.)

Nicholas Culpeper, 1653

The Greek physicians and their writings continued to inspire the medical world for many centuries exclusively. The Hippocratic Collection set the standard for the ancient civilised world, held sway throughout the Middle Ages, and still continues to influence it to-day in many ways. In Europe, during the Middle Ages, great advances were certainly made in surgery, and through the study of anatomy and physiology more definite knowledge was gained of the structure and functions of the human body, which led the way for the research that culminated in Harvey's great discovery of the circulation of the blood in the year 1628. Yet, in spite of these startling innovations, knowledge concerning psychological disorders and their treatment remained at a standstill. Conservatism retained the ancient theory of the wandering uterus as the cause of hysteria, and as late as the middle of the seventeenth century we find curious, and what seem to us to be superstitious and absurd, remedies being advised for the cure of Hysteria.

Thus in a book published in 1653, called *Pharmacopoeia Londonensis*, or the *London Dispensatory*, written by Nicholas Culpeper, who is described as "A Gent Student in Physick and Astrology, living in Spittle-fields near London," we find a detailed description of the accepted cure for Hysteria, which is given in full in a note at the end of this chapter, for the sake of its intrinsic interest as well as for the merit of the suggestion contained in the last sentence, "Neither is the womb often afflicted, but the head principally suffers with it."

This suggestion put forward by Culpeper stimulates sufficient curiosity to lead us to investigate what he has to say about curing the sufferings connected with the head, which we find necessarily include afflictions of the brain. Immediately we are faced with problems presented to the mind of a scientist, who was a Student in Astrology as well as in Physick. Medicines, frequently made from distilled herbs, were appropriated to various parts of the body, and mankind was grouped according to their prevalent "*humours*"—Choller, Blood, Melancholy, and Flem. Melancholy was naturally regarded as a disease connected with the brain, and it was accurately observed by early medical men that the larger number of these troubles would fluctuate in their severity rather than remain constant. This was also observed in connection with hysteria. On account of this variable characteristic they were thought to be associated with the changes of the moon in some way. Herbs that were named because of some real or fancied resemblance to this inconstant giver of light were prescribed for them, chief among which was the *lunaria*, or moon-wort; and in connection with this same observed periodicity, many conditions we should now group as nervous were termed *Lunatic Diseases*, or *Lunacy*.

Here, again, it was not the observation of facts where these old physicians went astray as much as in the *causes* to which they attributed the manifest symptoms. In the nervous diseases of women especially a clearly marked fluctuation is usually apparent, which may or may not coincide exactly with the phases of the moon, but which certainly corresponds with her own periodicity of menstruation, which, like the lunar month, is of twenty-eight days. Some physiologists maintain that an analogous rhythm may also be observed in men, but of a shorter span, this being one of twenty-one days only, against that of the woman's twenty-eight days. They believe also that "the possibility of men undergoing a monthly rhythm similar to that which women undergo is worth considering." (Harry Campbell, M.D., F.R.C.P., *Differences in the Nervous Organisation of Man and Woman*, H. K. Lewis, Ltd.)

Institution of Hydrotherapy

As yet, however, the real significance of the coincidence of one symptom and another condition which have been observed in the same person had not penetrated the minds of these physicians of yesterday. The latter half of the seventeenth century, however, saw a new form of therapy added to the resources of the medical man of the period, and also popularised the terminology of another emotional trouble. The new name to be found in the current literature of that day was "*the Vapours*," which had been known to Culpeper as the Vapours of Melancholy, its symptoms varying between those now usually identified with the lighter forms of hysteria on the one hand, and with those typical of melancholia on the other, although it was at the same time a fashionable pose to simulate its symptoms and to take the new cure which was found to be exceedingly diverting.

The remedy that was invented at the same time to cure or alleviate the condition was to order the patient a course of taking the waters, now called *hydro-therapy*, which still continues to enjoy a certain amount of popularity. A visit was paid to a fashionable watering-place—Tunbridge Wells, or, during the next century, Bath—where patients, as well as their jaded relations, found pleasant relief from the monotonous routine of home life. The change of air, change of scene, cheerful diversions and excitements of all descriptions, besides the supposed direct benefit conferred upon them through drinking the chalybeate waters, which were thought efficacious in cases of "cold chronical distempers, weak nerves, and bad digestion," according to a writer of the period.

This new health resort received Royal support. Catharine of Braganza, an unhappy lady, whom we may imagine, from what is now known about the causes of psycho-neuroses, must often have required cures or diversions of this kind, was a constant visitor at Tunbridge Wells, and by her presence made the place and the remedy equally fashionable. An interesting side-light upon the opinion of that time concerning this remedy is, however, to be found in the memories of Lord Boyle, quoted in *Highways and Byeways of Kent* (Walter Jerrold. Macmillan & Co.): "We are ordered down here commonly *pour la Maladie Imaginaire,* for the spirits and the melancholy, to which our whole Nation are too subject. The Diversions and Amusements of the Place send us home again *Chearfull,* and the Foggy Air of London with the Disappointments of Life, urge our Return the following year—The Water has a brackish taste never palatable."

Half a century later we find Mrs. "Blue-stocking" Montagu (*ibid.*) giving a more detailed description of the daily routine prescribed for those undergoing the cure: "So many glasses of water to be drunk, so many buttered rolls to be eaten, so many turns on the walk [the Pantiles, of course, is to be understood], so many miles to be gone in a post chaise or on horse-back, so much pains to be well, so much attention to be civil."

The popularity of Tunbridge Wells as a health resort waned, Bath followed as its rival, under the Regency, which in its turn was eclipsed by the glories of Brighton in the reign of George IV, when the attention of the public was called to the health-giving virtues of sea-water bathing. A relic of this once fashionable cure still survives in the Sea Water Dispensary in the Euston Road, London.

It is interesting to note how persistently these old remedies have retained the allegiance of medical men in the treatment of nervous diseases. We may still find one that recalls the method of Galen and Culpeper in the administration of Valerian, with its unpleasant taste and disagreeable smell, which is considered a specific drug for use in cases of hysteria and other neurotic conditions, especially in women. We also still hear of medical practitioners who recommend their patients who are suffering from neurotic disorders to visit some Spa or Hydro, at home or abroad, suggesting a sea-voyage, or telling them that it would be beneficial to find some new occupation which would act as a diversion of their thoughts from themselves or their troubles. The patient still eagerly carries out the doctor's orders, now as then. For a time the "nerves" or melancholy will be greatly improved, but upon the return home relapse as frequently occurs, which necessitates a fresh trip to some new health resort where the old conditions are once more left behind for the time being.

Introduction of Hypnotism Through Mesmer, 1734–1815

At the end of the eighteenth century another milestone was reached marking the course of the treatment of these disorders. Physicians on the Continent began to avail themselves of a process which, although dating back through many centuries in the East, had until this time received very little attention from Western nations, from the point of view of scientific medical investigation. This was

Hypnotism, which received new impetus from its celebrated exponent Mesmer, who explained his method as the action of a mysterious force or fluid, which was supposed to emanate from the operator upon the patient. The name which was then given to this form of treatment was *Mesmerism*, after the doctor who was the first to demonstrate its uses throughout Europe. For a long time this name was given to many variations of similar psychological treatments, which had an undoubted suggestive influence that effected the cure or alleviation of those who believed in its efficacy. But through its use in the hands of those who treated it as an exhibition merely of their own miraculous power over others, as it might be a side-show at a fair, it consequently fell into disrepute as the trick of a charlatan, which led to the medical profession in this country, as well as throughout the Continent of Europe, looking askance at all who wished to practise Mesmerism upon their patients and make use of it for legitimate scientific uses. We shall see exactly what effect this unwillingness to receive psychological methods of treating had during the next two centuries, when several pioneers were striving to advance existing knowledge concerning the psychological disorders and to introduce new ways of alleviating them.

It is interesting to note, however, that although very little actually remains of the treatment as practised by Mesmer, the idea that lay at the foundation of his belief in his ability to cure his patients is only too familiar to-day in numberless people who are dealing with patients of this description especially, although they probably have no realisation of the origin of their feeling about themselves and their patients, or its relation to Mesmerism. The expression which gives us a clue as to the connection between the former means of treatment and the present-day attitude of many nurses lies in these words, which we will all recognise as familiar enough: "*They take it out of oneself so!*" or, "*One is giving out all the time.*" Asked what "it" represents, one wonders if anyone could say, but it sounds like the mysterious fluid or power which was supposed to pass from the mesmerist to his patient. They certainly feel that they can and do influence their patients, and probably unconsciously link up this feeling, as well as the comfortable idea of power that it brings, with the records of miracles which are given in the Bible—miracles which, it must be remembered, happened in the East, where the influence of one mind over another has been known and used long before we had any conscious knowledge of its power, or thought of enlisting it in the service of medicine.

However, in spite of obstacles, the influence of Mesmer was soon felt spreading widely throughout Europe. Scientists, who were independent enough to act upon their own initiative, visited him, to observe for themselves the truth of the phenomena which were stated to result from the use of his method, as well as to make themselves masters of the technique.

The history of the development of Mesmerism and its growing application in medicine is one that is unusually interesting, since in it one may trace in the opposition which it encountered a typical instance of the hesitation of medical men in general to adopt new ideas, and their tendency to take for granted that an innovation must be either useless or, if effectual, unlawful. Consequent upon this opinion we find that those who tried to spread the use and knowledge of this new treatment were stringently forbidden to do so, and many were deprived of their posts in consequence of it. This recalls the treatment of mediæval scientists, who were usually supposed to be in league with the Devil, and might be condemned to be burnt at the stake, escaping this fate only by means of recantation of their heresy, which was their scientific discovery won through arduous research, like Galileo.

JOHN ELLIOTSON, 1791–1868

The pioneer in England to attempt the introduction of Mesmerism was John Elliotson, son of a Southwark chemist. He was born in 1791, and having received the sound foundation of a classical education, studied medicine in Edinburgh, where he took his M.D. His next step was to visit the most celebrated medical schools on the Continent, and returned eager to carry out further research, first at Cambridge and then in St. Thomas's and Guy's Hospitals. He returned from abroad keen to practise the new methods which he had learned, but was immediately confronted with serious obstacles. Opposition, if not direct hostility, was encountered from all sides. In 1817 he was appointed Assistant Physician to St. Thomas's Hospital, and Physician six years later, but found it extremely difficult to gain permission to give clinical lectures. These, however, when given, were received with much interest. To Elliotson also we owe the modern use of quinine in large doses, the demonstration of the specific use of iodide of potassium, and the value of iron in chorea.

Another medical innovation that must be connected with the name of Elliotson is the use of the stethoscope in England, which he adopted directly after the publication of Laennec's work on the subject (*Hypnotism*, by J. Milne Bramwell. William Rider & Son, 1913). Its use, nevertheless, at first drew nothing but abuse and ridicule from his professional colleagues, and a senior Fellow of the College of Physicians pointed out the folly of "carrying a piece of wood into a sick-room." The general opinion seemed to be that nothing was to be learned by its use, and even if there were the disease could in no way be treated any better for the knowledge so gained.

Institution of University College Hospital

In 1831 Elliotson received the appointment of Professor of the Practice of Medicine at University College, and it is in connection with this post that his chief work was carried out in attempting to demonstrate the value of mesmerism to medicine. University College Hospital was instituted mainly at Elliotson's solicitation, and here he pursued this so far little explored science with signal success, attracting so large a concourse of students that he was obliged to mesmerise patients in the lecture theatre instead of in the wards. However, great as this work was, it was destined to receive a serious check, and from no other source than the Council of University College itself. In the year 1838 they passed a resolution that "the Hospital Committee be instructed to take such steps as they shall deem most advisable to prevent the practice of mesmerism or animal magnetism in future within the hospital." The result of this decision was that Elliotson was ordered to cease mesmerising his patients. He thereupon resigned his appointment and never entered the hospital nor the college again. The restriction was a severe blow to his work, and he felt the decree unfair, since the majority of the members of the Council had never witnessed his experiments nor discussed the method with him.

Another violent attack was made upon this ardent pioneer in 1846, when his turn came to deliver the Harveian Oration; still, it did not deter him from taking the application of Mesmerism as the subject of the address. Earnestly he besought his hearers to investigate this new method for themselves, and not to repudiate it without careful research, "if they cared for truth, their own dignity, and the good of mankind."

Three years earlier Elliotson and his followers had started a journal, called the *Zoist,* for the collection of information respecting cerebral anatomy and mesmerism. It appeared quarterly, and continued to do so for thirteen years, until the end of 1855. Elliotson himself contributed many articles to its pages describing various uses of the method. In them he explained its anæsthetic properties during amputations of the thigh, leg, arm, breast, and also postulated cure or alleviation in cases of insanity, epilepsy, hystero-epilepsy, hysteria, stammering, neuralgia, asthma, torticollis, headache, functional affections of the heart, rheumatism, and other diseases could be obtained by this method, and that mesmerism was especially useful in hysteria and other functional nervous disorders. These diseases, he pointed out, were seldom understood and often received treatment that was worse than useless in the practice of blistering, bleeding, and salivation. He also made the assertion that was startling for those days, that hysteria was not only confined to women, but also frequently occurred in males.

We must, in addition to the work already described, remember the name of John Elliotson as one who introduced new views in the now familiar sphere of child welfare and the medical treatment of children. He pointed out that many of the conditions usually attributed to *naughtiness* were due to ill-health, "that convulsions sometimes arose from overwork, and terror was no uncommon cause of nervous affections."

The work commenced in England by John Elliotson was followed by Esdaile, James Braid, and many others. The uses to which the method was first put were extended, and the technique itself underwent some modifications in course of time. Braid at length suggested that it should be called *Hypnotism* instead of Mesmerism, and defined the term as *the induction of nervous sleep.* With the work of this physician, however, the method reached its highest point of popularity in this country, and after his death in 1860 psycho-therapy practically ceased in England until some years had elapsed, when a revival from a fresh source, introducing a new method, took place.

THE SCHOOL AT NANCY. DR. A. A. LIÉBEAULT. BERNHEIM.

The interest in hypnotism, nevertheless, maintained a steady increase in Europe, one of the outstanding figures in the movement being Dr. Liébeault, of Nancy (b. 1823). At first his work was chiefly among the French peasants, but his fame spread, and patients as well as students from all parts began to flock to attend his clinic for purposes of cure or study. In 1882 he cured an obstinate case of sciatica of six years' duration, whom a colleague, by name Bernheim, had treated in vain, which aroused the incredulity and afterwards the admiration of that doctor. He became a keen student of Liébeault's methods and his lifelong friend, publishing two years later an account of work done at the clinic at Nancy. The first part of the work was called *De la Suggestion*, the second, *La Thérapeutic Suggestive*, which appeared in 1886.

As we may infer from the titles of these two books, a new element had now appeared in the curative method—the use of suggestion allied to hypnotism, or rather it was administered during the hypnotic sleep. No drugs were prescribed for the treatment of patients, and Liébeault would explain to his patients that he neither possessed nor exercised any supernatural power, all he did was quite simple, and it was open to scientific investigation of every description.

The term *School of Nancy* is connected equally with the names of Liébeault and Bernheim, since it was through the writings of the latter that the "good father Liébeault," as he was called, became famous. Otherwise his ministry would probably have escaped general recognition, since he was not the type of man to seek personal fame, being interested rather in the cure of his patients, the poor sick folk who could gain no other help for their many troubles, which indeed were of many kinds, which extended beyond the scope of ordinary medicine. It is interesting to note that Bernheim made the discovery that his hospital patients were more readily influenced by suggestion under hypnosis than were his private patients, owing to their greater susceptibility to suggestion and their lack of critical faculty. (*Die Medizin der Gegenwart in Selbstdarstellungen.* Sigmund Freud. Felix Meiner, Leipzig, 1925.) Liébeault used to inform his students that his nervous and hysterical patients were the most difficult cases, the reason for this will become clear to the reader by the explanations of neurotic disorder and the part it plays in the life of the patient in subsequent chapters of this book.

Salpêtrière School. Charcot.

The second medical school of repute for the treatment of psycho-neuroses, which flourished at the same time as that of Nancy, was instituted at Salpêtrière by Charcot and the students whom he gathered round him there to learn his methods. While resembling the teaching of Liébeault in many respects, it differed widely in others. There also nervous diseases of all types received treatment and improved under it, chief among which should be mentioned hysterical paralysis and contractures, epilepsy and many forms of insanity.

As a teacher he sought to spread his methods more keenly than Liébeault, and he had made the hospital of Salpêtrière the goal of his ambitions while still a young man. In the hall in which he used to deliver his famous "*Leçons du Mardi*" hung the portrait of the celebrated Citizen Pinel, causing the poor insane of Salpêtrière to be delivered of their chains. A rare and valuable intimacy was allowed between Charcot and his pupils, who became almost members of his family, were welcomed frequently at his house, and enjoyed many personal discussions with the great master. (*Charcot.* Sigmund Freud. Collected Papers. Vol. I. Hogarth Press.)

Charcot's chief work, perhaps, concerned discoveries upon the nature and manifestations of hysteria, which he regarded as almost entirely an *hereditary disease*, a view that more recent investigations have questioned. He also applied himself to prove that certain conditions which had been ascribed to alcoholic or lead poisoning were hysterical, and that hysteria was far more common among men than was generally believed, especially among those belonging to the working classes. Another field of Charcot's work concerned the re-education of public opinion in regard to the usual sneering attitude adopted towards the woman who suffered from hysteria, for he "threw the whole weight of his authority on the side of the reality and objectivity of the hysterical phenomena." Thus Charcot, by this attempt, repeated on a small scale the act of liberation commemorated in the picture of Pinel, which adorned the lecture-hall of Salpêtrière.

As we have already mentioned, Charcot was not only a great physician, he was almost more renowned as a teacher. In connection with him and his school we should always bear in mind at least two names, which stand out with conspicuous lustre from among the ranks of his many famous pupils. These are Sigmund Freud and Janet. But while the latter continued to follow in the footsteps of his master and carry on the work of hypnotism and suggestion in France, Freud was destined to revolutionise both the theory and treatment of functional Nervous Diseases after his return to Vienna.

Sigmund Freud, b. 1856

It is especially interesting in studying the contribution made by Sigmund Freud to medical science concerning psycho-neuroses to observe to what extent he derived the ideas which led to his discovery, *Psycho-analysis*, from others, and to notice how far other methods of psycho-therapy, now used by medical men who abuse and repudiate Freudian teaching, have actually been constructed from them, although in many cases totally without any acknowledgment of their distinguished parentage.

Freud was born on May 6, 1856, in Mähren, a little town in what is now known as Czechoslovakia. When he was four years old the family moved to Vienna, where later he matriculated and entered the University. At first he felt no ambition to devote his life and energies to medicine, but finally took this step, having become interested in the study of the Nervous System while in the physiological laboratory of Ernst Brücke. The road then led through this laboratory to the study of cranial anatomy, and eventually to that of the *Diseases of the Nervous System.* In those days this remained still an almost unexplored territory, and Freud tells himself in his autobiography, published in the series *Die Medizin der Gegenwart in Selbstdarstellungen,* that in these days little was known about such remote diseases, and even celebrated authorities in Vienna would diagnose Neurasthenia as Cerebral Tumour.

With the ambition before him of becoming a specialist in nervous diseases, Freud began seriously to equip himself for this profession. He gained a teaching appointment at the University, through the interest of Ernst Brücke, to which was a travelling stipend, which enabled him to visit Paris in order to study at Salpêtrière, in 1885, as one of Charcot's pupils. Whilst there this enthusiastic young doctor undertook the arduous labour of translating the already published medical works of Charcot, and was thereupon admitted into his intimate circle of friends and pupils.

The work at Salpêtrière which attracted the greatest interest from Freud was that connected with Hysteria in all its forms, including information concerning the genuineness and constancy of hysterical phenomena, the frequency of occurrence of Hysteria in men, the production of hysterical paralysis and contractures during hypnoses, and the knowledge that these artificial conditions showed the same characteristics as those which arose spontaneously, often in consequence of some trauma (accident).

On his way back to Vienna, Freud spent some time in Berlin under Baginski, in order to study the common nervous diseases of children, since Kassowitz, who was director of a public hospital for children in Vienna, had promised to allow him to open a ward for the nervous diseases of children on his return. Several years later, in 1891, Freud made use of the knowledge gained from these sources to publish several important papers upon the cerebral paralysis of children.

In the autumn of 1886 Freud settled down in Vienna and married. It was due to this occurrence that he was not able to carry out research that would have also connected his name with the discovery of the anæsthetic properties of cocaine in minor surgery. His monograph on the subject, *Über die Coca pflanze* (Verlag. Franz Deutike), is little known and now generally unobtainable, whereas the discoverer of this valuable anæsthetic is usually considered to be Carl Koller, now in New York.

On his return to Vienna, eager to spread the information that he had gained during his sojourn in Paris, Freud was confronted with opposition from his older and more conservative colleagues, similar to that which met Elliotson in London many years previously. Especially did his statement concerning the frequency of Hysteria in men call forth ridicule, although he was able to demonstrate the characteristic symptoms in several patients with whom he confronted his opponents.

In those days the would-be specialist in psycho-neuroses had only three resources at his command. The first possibility was to send patients to take cures at Spas or watering-places, yet this was scarcely a satisfactory expedient from a financial standpoint for the physician. Besides this, the other two forms of treatment that remained were electro-therapy and hypnosis. Freud made an exhaustive study of the handbook written by the expert W. Erb, but was forced, through experience gained by means of experiment with the methods described, to reach the conclusion that success which was achieved by these means was usually brought about through the influence of suggestion on the part of the doctor and the readiness on the part of the patient to receive these suggestions.

Finally, Freud laid aside his electric batteries and once more devoted himself to a protracted study of the phenomena of hypnosis and the use of suggestion during the hypnoid state, as well as another method which had been mentioned to him by a colleague in Vienna before he had gone to Paris. He had become familiar with the combination of suggestion and hypnosis whilst watching the work of Charcot, and in the summer of 1889 he took advantage of the vacation to visit Nancy, there to perfect his technique with observation of the methods of Dr. Liébeault, as well as to study the remarkable experiments that were being carried out by Bernheim upon his patients in hospital. Upon this journey he took with him an especially interesting case of a young girl suffering from hysteria, to see whether Bernheim could advance her cure farther than he had been able to do, but without success.

It was this failure to gain complete recovery of health for patients gifted with a high degree of intelligence which led Freud to feel the necessity of finding some other method of cure that should prove effectual when others failed. With this aim in view he set himself to investigate afresh the scientific information which he had been given by his friend some years previously. This colleague was Dr. Josef Breuer, a family physician in Vienna. Among his large practice he had been conducting the case of a young girl, severely afflicted with a number of psychogenic symptoms. He had begun by treating her with hypnosis, but in course of the treatment made the remarkable discovery that led to his formulation of a new theory of the causes of hysteria and a fresh means of bringing relief to the sufferers from this disease, even were actual cure not practicable.

The new treatment which had thus been accidentally brought to light was this: that to allow the patient to speak freely about all that came into the mind concerning the cause of the illness, or anything else that occurred to her during the hypnosis, as well as in the waking state, would cause great relief of mental tension. The improvement that Breuer noticed in the mental condition in his first patient from this method was so striking that he continued the experiment upon others, meeting with similar success in each case. It will be noticed that the procedure of this treatment differed essentially from that which had formerly been in use allied with hypnosis for the treatment of hysteria, in that the patient told what had been the cause of the trouble while the doctor listened; whereas, formerly, the patient listened during the hypnosis to suggestions concerning the recovery from the distressing symptom which were made by the physician. The result which was achieved thus, the relief of the patient's mind through talking of past worries and anxieties, led to the theory which Breuer postulated by means of these discoveries, concerning the origin of the hysterical symptom as well as the onset of the trouble, that some crisis in the life of the patient had aroused intense emotion which at the time was unable to find any adequate discharge. The patient therefore continued to seek some outlet for this pent-up emotion by means of a constant repetition of the original scene or some detail connected with it, although the relation between them may have been entirely forgotten by the patient, or may, indeed, never have been realised. When it became possible to give the patient an adequate discharge for this stored emotion, as well as to bring back into conscious memory the forgotten link between the original traumatic event and the present symptom, cure or alleviation of the nervous trouble is brought about.

As we have mentioned already, Freud was acquainted with this discovery of Breuer's before his visit to Paris, and had, indeed, attempted to interest Charcot in this new method, but he had met with little success, and temporarily had been obliged to set it on one side for further investigation when occasion should allow. The inadequacy of electrotherapy as a curative method, however, provided the stimulus that was needful, and led Freud back to renewed research along the lines of Breuer's innovation. For a time they worked in collaboration, and in 1895 published a book describing the method and the theories deduced from its use as a curative method. This work, *Studien über Hysterie,* was received with coldness by the members of the medical profession in Vienna, which was a matter of considerable disappointment to the elder of its joint authors, Breuer, and probably was an important factor in his wish to abandon further investigations in this direction a few years later. The work that had already been done was nevertheless momentous, and made a stepping-stone to wider discoveries before many years had passed. Breuer called his method of treatment *catharsis*, or the *cathartic treatment,* and the discharge of emotion obtained by this means *abreaction.* This method was successfully revived in Germany during the Great War, for the treatment of soldiers suffering from shell-shock, by Dr. Ernst Simmel, who is now directing a Sanatorium for patients suffering from psycho-neuroses at Schloss Tegel, on the outskirts of Berlin, although the method now principally in use there is Freud's derivative from it, *psycho-analysis.*

Originally it had been the *symptom* which had gained the chief attention of these two physicians, but Freud became unwilling to confine his research to this factor alone. He was determined, if possible, to carry the investigation still farther, and to ascertain the cause of the disease and the reason why one type of symptom should have been chosen rather than another. It was this desire on the part of the younger man which became the manifest cause of their separation. The elder brought forward the reasons that he had neither the time nor the inclination to give to research of this description, and preferred to devote himself as before to general practice, as well as the fact that he hesitated to probe farther into the roots of the psychogenesis of hysteria, feeling that they had gone far enough. But behind these reasons that were given it is difficult not to feel that the disapprobation of the majority of the medical profession of Vienna had not cast the die of his decision, although he may not have realised that this had been so himself. The younger man, however, was by no means willing to rest content with the progress that had been already made, but was anxious as his companion was reluctant to press eagerly forward and establish the new theories as a formulated system, upon which it would be possible to base a theory of the origin of hysteria itself, as well as a method of cure, which should prove reliable to achieve success in the hitherto inaccessible cases of hysteria, besides other forms of nervous disease, in which hypnosis and suggestion were not beneficial.

This collaboration between these two friends ceased, and Freud continued his work alone. He soon found important elements in common among his patients which enabled him to postulate the theory that the cause of hysteria, as well as the origin of the symptom, were generally provided by some conflict or disturbance in the emotional or love life of the patient that may also be inferred from the theories of the ancient physician, and those who came after them, although the connection had hitherto not been made clear between them.

To Freud, nevertheless, this came at first as a startling revelation, such as it also proved subsequently when introduced to the rest of the medical world, who opposed it with the utmost hostility. He afterwards recollected, however, that he had met with corroborative evidence not only from Breuer himself, but also from Charcot and Chrobak, as well as among the writings of Galen, Plato, and Havelock Ellis. Books of the last-mentioned authority were already beginning to attract considerable attention at that time, and these proofs that another had found the same facts as himself along a different line of research gave welcome support to his own discoveries, although these certainly met with little interest from his medical colleagues, but rather open contempt and animosity.

These new theories made their original appearance, after the book written with Breuer, in the pages of French and Viennese medical journals, although they were afterwards collected and published in book form; and in the year 1900 Freud's first important work came from the press, *The Interpretation of Dreams,* which has since been translated into more than a dozen different languages. This volume set out to demonstrate the great significance he had found in the patient's dreams for the understanding of the neurotic symptom and the origin of the onset of the disorder. The volume also contained a description of the theory of the Unconscious Mind, which represents a method of thinking rather than a spatial division of the brain, in which may be located many desires and impulses that had failed to find expression or satisfaction in our childhood, whence they are always striving to escape and win a direct or indirect gratification in the psycho-neurosis.

Since Freud had continued his work alone, he had made

several significant changes in this new treatment, foremost among which was the disuse of hypnotism as the vehicle of the method, first, because he had found that many people could not be hypnotised, and, secondly, he had discovered other more direct ways of bringing into consciousness the traumatic incident that had been the origin of the trouble. Subsequently it became clear to him that in forms other than hysteria it was necessary to work with other aims in view than merely the finding of the emotional crisis, as the cause of the trouble had not been one event alone, but rather a great number having a cumulative effect. In other cases the cause had been traced to an emotional relationship between the child and the parents in the early years of the particular individual which had led to these unfortunate consequences. He retained the reclining position as an assistance to the necessary condition of relaxation of the mind, and instructed his patients to say freely all the thoughts that came into their minds. He found that this, practised without reservation, eventually gave the same results as had the former talking under hypnosis, with the additional benefit that the patient was also aware at the time of what was being said, without it being necessary to give instructions during the sleeping state that it should be remembered when awake. This improved method Freud called *Free-association,* while to the method itself he gave the name of *Psycho-analysis.*

One book swiftly followed another, and more valuable theories were disclosed to assist with the understanding of that dark realm, the human mind. The three fundamental theories upon which the psycho-analytic method has been built up are these:

1. *Repression,* which implies *amnesia,* or the forgetting of painful incidents or emotions, which thus constructs a barrier of defence between us and these experiences of childhood that we do our best to obliterate.

2. *The Unconscious Mind,* by which is postulated the division of the mental life into two sections, the one conscious, with which we are familiar and in daily contact, the other unconscious, divided from the conscious mind by the thick curtain or barrier we call repression, in which remain unchanged the primitive impulses and wishes of childhood.
3. *The Importance of the Emotional Life of Childhood,* and essentially the part played by love and hate, together with the effective relationship between children and their parents, brothers, and sisters.

For about ten years Freud continued to work alone, but eventually his books found their way into other countries, and earnest disciples sought him out in Vienna to learn more about these discoveries and new methods. Gradually a small circle of devoted followers grouped themselves round him, most of whom have remained loyal. Some, it is true, have been separated by death, and a very few, comparatively, withdrew from the little company to form groups of their own, differing in some ways from the teaching of their master, or to concentrate upon one detail of psycho-analytic theory in isolation from the rest.

One of the most conspicuous of the young men who gathered round Freud in these early days, in the light of subsequent events, was Dr. C. G. Jung, from the psychiatric school at Zürich, who for many years was the editor of the first psycho-analytic journal. Divergent views finally separated him from Freud, and he, in course of time, withdrew from the newly formed Psycho-analytical Society to form a school of his own in Zürich, to which he gave the name of *Analytical Psychology.*

In 1909 Freud was invited to give a week's lectures at the Clark University, Worcester, Massachusetts, during the celebrations of their twentieth anniversary; and following this visit translations of Freud's most important works appeared in English, from the pen of Dr. A. A. Brill, of the Bronx Hospital and Columbia University, so that it at last became possible for those who could not read German to profit by this new teaching.

Other Schools of Psycho-therapy

The derivatives of psycho-analysis deserve some mention, since some of them emphasise one or other detail of Freudian doctrine, or have been formed in partial opposition to it, although clearly showing the sources whence they have sprung. However interesting or important each theory may prove in itself, all nevertheless seem to lose weight should one come to be regarded as the sole root for every form of neurosis. Several different schools have obviously taken their pattern from the original discoveries of Freud, and many of the men who are now leaders of separate groups were once his pupils. First let us mention the *Zurich School of Analytical Psychology*, with Dr. C. G. Jung as its founder and director. Similar in many ways, and based upon the Freudian conception, it has given a different value to the idea of symbolism in the human mind as shown in dreams, phantasies, and neurotic symptoms. Jung also abandons the search for the actual experience, the forgotten incident, to investigate the phantasy and allegory, giving supreme value to the abstract idea, the impersonal and unhistoric, rather than to the recollections of individual experience. His chief theories upon which he constructs the origin of neurosis are *the wish to return to the mother* and *the struggle for rebirth.*

Jung's separation from the Psycho-analytical Society (see note at the end of this chapter) was followed soon afterwards, in 1913, by that of another former pupil of Freud, Alfred Adler, who wished principally to stress the importance of the individual's struggle for power as the foundation of neurosis or the neurotic tendency. He has given the name of *Individual Psychology* to his theories, and attempts to show that all human beings have but one aim in life, be they male or female, "*to be an entire man,*" and that the wish that forms the mainspring of life is to gain supreme power as a compensation for some real or imaginary organ inferiority, which leaves the person with a feeling of incompleteness.

Wilhelm Stekel, another former student of Freud, has also broken away from the psycho-analytic group to develop the theory of *universal criminality of neurotic persons,* which he calls the aggressive impulse, the desire to cherish and develop their own "*beloved ego*" at the expense of the whole universe.

Besides these distinct groups which have arisen from Freudian discoveries, several well-known medical men in England and America, calling themselves psycho-analysts, or psychologists, have evolved variants of their own; but the differences consist chiefly in pruning away some portion of the original teaching which is not to their liking, or which does not meet with general approval, for which they have substituted a more palatable alternative. Many have also remained at the very early stages of psycho-analytic research and the first developments of the technique, not troubling to keep pace with the later additions and investigations, although they do not hesitate to reproach Freud for leaving so much ground uncovered, an idea which has arisen in their minds mainly because they have not been able or willing to read his more recent works in which these subjects are discussed.

Psycho-therapy received an urgent dynamic from the necessity which arose of dealing with the problem of large numbers of cases of traumatic neuroses after and during the Great War. In Germany, France, and England various methods were used both in the temporary hospitals behind the lines as well as in the permanent hospitals at the Base, or in clinics away from the fighting area. Electro-therapy, hypnotism, and more active forms of suggestion and "persuasion" were used, and rarely something that more or less resembled psycho-analysis and the cathartic treatment. Several books were published on the subject giving detailed descriptions of cases, treatment, and results; but this question will come again under discussion in the last chapter of this book, devoted to the nervous diseases of men and boys, among which will be included shell-shock and allied psychogenic troubles.

Electro-therapy

Electrical treatment has been used for many years with beneficial results for some forms of nerve troubles, including hysterical contractures and paralysis, but the actual curative principle may, it is true, be effected by direct or indirect suggestion spoken or implied by the skilled operator and the co-operation of the suggestibility of the patient, as much as that arising from the use of the electric current itself. It is an interesting sign of an increase in the general belief in psycho-therapy that the practitioners of many other kinds of treatment are incorporating some form of psychotherapy or suggestion with their own methods, such as the use of electric currents, massage, and the like. This suggestion may be direct or indirect, and it is often carried out by those who have very little knowledge concerning its use, the cases in which it might be suitable or the reverse, nor how it should be carried out, which is unfortunate. In reading some books brought out in the Military Medical Manuals Series, to be found in the list of those that may be read in connection with our last chapter, and from actual experience of cases treated at that time, the use of the electric battery seems often to have been extended past legitimate means of medical or scientific use, forcing patients through fear or pain to believe or to say that their conditions were improved, so that they might escape further application of this refinement of torture.

S. Weir-Mitchell, 1830–1914. Weir-Mitchell Treatment, Rest-Cures

Before concluding this chapter on the development of knowledge concerning the neurotic disorders it is necessary to mention two distinguished American medical men: Weir-Mitchell, a celebrated physician whose name is familiar to every nurse in connection with the special treatment that bears his name for the cure of nervous exhaustion and debility and also with rest-cures; the other, G. W. Crile, a surgeon who has taken the psychological aspect of his patients into consideration in a remarkable way, that shall presently be described. The trained nurse is associated more particularly, perhaps, with the Weir-Mitchell treatment and with rest-cures than with many others, since she is so often put in sole charge to carry it out and may be sent away with the patient for the purpose, unless a nursing-home is advised, in which case also she will still be intimately concerned with the ultimate success of the cure. It usually consists, as we all know, of a prolonged rest in bed, abundant diet, commencing with milk only. Separation from home and friends is imperative, no letters may be written or received, nor are visits allowed. No occupations break the monotony of the first few weeks, except that massage is given daily, this and meals form the only exertion that confronts the patient, so that complete rest may be achieved. In a recent description of the method to be found in the seventh edition of *Practical Nursing*, by Cuff and Pugh, we find the significant words, "occasionally psycho-therapy in the form of suggestion is employed," but this was not one of the original components of the treatment as prescribed by Weir-Mitchell himself, who relied upon the physiological factors of food and rest alone to restore the health of his patients.

The great difficulty in carrying out the essential of this treatment is actually to procure *rest* for the patient, not only of the body, which may be simple enough, but also of the mind, without which the former will generally be unavailing. In some cases of nervous exhaustion or the effects of over-work, it is true, physical rest may be all that is needed to re-establish mental balance, but for any form of long-standing neurosis mental rest from worry or anxiety is by far the most important factor. This, nevertheless, is more difficult to procure. Absence from home and relatives may be a step towards a resolution of the problem, but it usually has but a temporary effect. Once the ordinary routine of daily life and the difficult conditions which caused the trouble in the first place have to be faced afresh, the symptoms are frequently revived and a renewal of the treatment becomes necessary.

How the nurse may help to alleviate the real troubles of her patients, whom she has in her care for rest-cures, will be described later on in this book; but to enable them to maintain permanent recovery is always a difficult problem, since the situation of the greatest moment often lies in some family relationship or unwished-for environment, from which it is hard to escape except through the expedient of illness.

W. G. Crile, b. 1864, Anoci-Association

To Crile we owe much of our information about the effects of "*shock*" upon the recuperative power of the patient. He made special research upon the psychological effect of surgical operations, and studied ways in which post-operative shock might be minimised or avoided, particularly in those connected with the removal of the thyroid gland, which were recognised by him as especially closely associated with the mental or nervous disturbance of the patient. His method, called Anoci-Association, of anæsthetising each layer of tissue before incisions were made, in order to prevent painful stimuli reaching the brain, although the patient was under the influence of a general anæsthetic at the time, was a new advance in the conceptions of surgery, which showed a recognition that the psychological factors in the shock suffered by the patient were as important as the physiological components, which heretofore had been the only considerations of the surgeon.

EMIL COUÉ. AUTO-SUGGESTION

A few years ago the treatment of Coué for those suffering from many kinds of ailment was in the forefront of popularity, and Auto-suggestion made a wide appeal among a certain section of invalids, because it seemed to them a novelty and combined interest with the feeling that one was curing oneself. Auto-suggestion was therefore attractive to those who liked to feel their own power over themselves, although they quite overlooked the fact that in the first place the suggestion that this was possible had come from another, and was still hetero-suggestion in spite of the illusion to the contrary.

The little formula, which became a byword, *Every day and in every way I become better and better*, was indeed eventually inclined to bring a smile to the lips of many; but it has waned of late, other popular slogans, such as Eat More Fruit and Get the Brown Bread Habit, have taken its place to a great extent. Since the death of the inventor of this panacea for so many human complaints we do not hear so much of the wonders wrought by this means, although the Coué-Ortan Institute Limited continues to exist in London. It is interesting to observe that France has remained faithful to the influence of suggestion in many different forms, which leads us to suppose that the method must be peculiarly suitable to the national temperament and mentality.

Occupation-therapy

During the war Occupation-therapy enjoyed a certain vogue, and several special hospitals connected with wounded and shell-shocked soldiers made use of this as their main curative principle. In some cases it was effectual, but it is difficult to determine to what extent we can regard the cures as being permanent, or if they are more of the nature of a temporary alleviation. It is frequently impossible to keep in touch with the patients to know what the subsequent history may be; but it would seem that the result is often the same as after rest-cures, that a fresh difficulty arising in life, or a recurrence of an old one, will provide a renewal of the nervous debility or some special symptom, and once more the patient is returned to medical care, and one form of treatment will be tried after another without conspicuous success.

We shall have more to say about the underlying principles of the treatment in our last chapter, and will refer the reader to this section for further details.

The best-known hospitals where Occupation-therapy was used during and after the war were in Scotland and Golders Green, but they were found not to be the great success that had been hoped, and were closed after a short existence.

By means of this brief survey we may see the gradual progress by which present-day theories of the cause and effect of psycho-neuroses have been built up. How different centuries and the various countries of Europe, as well as Asia and America, have contributed their quota to the total knowledge which is now available on the subject for those who are anxious to seek it.

Many books have been written upon the causes of the

neuroses, which include descriptions of various kinds of physiological and psychological treatment to be carried out by the physician for the assistance of these patients. Yet, in these nervous diseases particularly, the nurse is an important factor in the success of the cure, which seems to indicate that the time has now come when the nursing of these cases should also undergo some investigation, and that the part she has to play in this great work of healing the nervously sick requires both description and explanation.

NOTE A TO CHAPTER I

FROM CULPEPER'S "PHARMACOPOEIA LONDONENSIS." CHAPTER VII, PAGE 310.

"A Key to Galen's Method of Physick."
Of Medicines appropriated to the Womb.

These, Physitians call Hystericals, and to avoid multiplicity of words, take them in this discourse under that notion.

. . . . .

As for the nature of the Womb, it seems to be much like the nature of the Brain and Stomach, for experience teacheth that it is delighted with sweet and Aromatical medicines and flies from their contraries.

For example, A Woman being troubled with the Fits of the Mother, which is drawing of the Womb upwards, apply sweet things, as Civit, or the like, to the place of Conception, it draws it down again, but apply stinking things to the nose as Assofœtida, or the like, it expels it from it and sends it down to its proper place.

Again, Sometimes the Womb of a Woman falls out, in such cases, sweet scents applied to the Nose, and stinking things to the privy passage, reduces it to its proper place again, and this made some Physitians of Opinion that the Womb of a Woman was capable of the sence of smelling. For my part I believe nothing less; only it doth it by apropriation to that part of the Body, for the Stomach also is offended with stinking things, not because it smells them, but because they are obnoxious to that part of the body, judg the like by the Womb; it is offended by stinking things, and strengthened by sweet; for smell is one of the Touch-stones by which Nature trieth what is convenient for itself; yet, that the Womb hath much affinity with the Head is most certain, and undeniable by this argument, Because most Cephalick Medicines conduce to the cure of Diseases in the Womb, neither is the Womb often afflicted, but the Head principally suffers with it.

NOTE B TO CHAPTER I

International Psycho-analytical Society

The beginnings of this Society lay in private meetings of a number of young medical men who gathered round Freud in his house in Vienna as early as 1902, for the purpose of learning, practising, and spreading knowledge of psycho-analysis. The first Psycho-analytical Congress was held at Salzburg, 1908, when the Vienna and Zurich Schools were united. Groups of the Society, their aim being still that of the first private circle in Vienna, are to be found in Vienna, Budapest, Zurich, Berlin, Holland, London, Paris, India, Moscow, Japan and New York, while its members number between three and four hundred.

It has five Institutes with Out-patient Clinics and teaching departments in Vienna, Berlin, London, The Hague, and Frankfort, and six journals, three published in Vienna, one in London, one in New York, and one in Paris.

BIBLIOGRAPHY

List of books that may be studied in connection with Chapters I, II, and III, giving further details of the growth of knowledge concerning the treatment of the psycho-neuroses and their causes, including Applied Psychology. The books are shown in chronological order of publication where possible. It will be understood that only a few representative works of some writers on these subjects have been chosen as being of special value to the nurse in the fulfilment of her duties.

1653. *Pharmacopoeia Londonensis*, or the *London Dispensatory*, by Nicholas Culpeper.

1909. *Selected Papers on Hysteria and Other Psychoneuroses*, by Prof. Dr. Sigmund Freud, LL.D., trans. A. A. Brill, M.D., Ph.B.

1913. *Hypnotism*, by J. Milne Bramwell, M.B., C.M.

1914. *Psychopathology of Everyday Life*, by Prof. Dr. Sigmund Freud, trans. A. A. Brill, M.D., Ph.B.

1916. *Mental Nursing*, by W. H. B. Stoddart, M.D., F.R.C.P.

1917. *Collected Papers upon Analytical Psychology*, by C. G. Jung, M.D., LL.D.

1918. *Psychology of the Unconscious*, by Dr. C. G. Jung.

1918. *The Neurotic Constitution*, by Dr. Alfred Adler.

1918. *Psychology of Insanity*, by Bernard Hart, M.D.

1920. *Treatment of the Neuroses*, by Ernest Jones, M.D.

1921. *The Beloved Ego*, by Dr. Wilhelm Stekel.

1921. *Introduction to Psychology*, by Susan Brierly, M.A.

1922. *Technique of Psycho-analysis*, by David Forsyth, M.D., D.Sc., F.R.C.P.

1925. *Outlines of Psychiatry*, by William A. White, M.D.

1925. *Psychology for Nurses*, by Mary Chadwick, S.R.N.

1927. *Practical Nursing* (7th Edition), by Herbert E. Cuff, M.D., F.R.C.S., and W. T. Gordon Pugh, M.D., B.C.

1927. *A Survey*: The Development of the Psycho-analytical Theory of the Psychoses, 1894–1926, by John Rickman, M.D.

1928. *A Short History of Medicine*, by Charles Singer, M.A., M.D., D.Litt., F.R.C.P.

1928. *Nervous and Mental Diseases for Nurses*, by Irving J. Sands, M.D.

1929. *A B C of Psychology*, by C. K. Ogden.

1930. *Don't be Tired*, by Dr. Peter Schmidt, trans. by Mary Chadwick.

CHAPTER II

HYSTERIA AND ITS CHIEF FORMS

Its Characteristic Forms and Symptoms
Methods of Treatment
The Part Played by the Nurse in the Course of the Illness

Before we are in a position to discuss the chief points of modern nursing methods to apply to patients suffering from neurotic disorders, using the knowledge that recent investigations of the causes and meaning of these serious troubles has placed at our disposal, it is necessary to have a clear picture in our mind what the trouble may actually represent from the patient's point of view, and not only from that of the onlooker, who has not yet been let into the secrets which have led to this state of affairs.

In choosing *Hysteria* as our starting-point we are not only retracing the steps by which the understanding of these strange states has evolved, but also representing that section of psycho-neuroses which is probably most extensive, when we consider its many branches, and one which will need the services of the nurse more extensively than many others, which often do not include any bodily symptoms or injuries that require special ministrations to need her presence. The treatment of such cases will then involve merely the patient and the physician to effect the cure.

The nurse in charge of the nerve case occupies a position of great importance, and yet one that is extremely difficult. Many doctors still do not realise the need for psychological treatment for these patients, and prescribe for them only rest, nourishing food, sedatives, and the personality of the nurse, who is to "strengthen the will of the patient," and in fact do all that is necessary to cause the patient to "pull him or herself together."

However, each year adds to the number of medical men who are realising that disorders arising from origins within the mind must be cured by treatment which is comparable with the cause, and are making use of some variety of psychotherapeutics. In such cases, naturally, the nurse finds that her burden of responsibility is lightened. Her knowledge of the mental picture of the disorder and the course of the illness is not only of great assistance in her own work, but she may often contribute largely to the success of the cure through supplying data by her observations that may be of value to the doctor as corroborating material he has obtained first-hand from the patient. There are also a few nursing-homes and larger institutions in Great Britain, Europe, and America where psychological treatment is being used extensively, and the nurses are being trained to understand this branch of medical service for the treatment of neurotic and mental disease, as they already receive thorough instruction in the nursing of medical and surgical cases.

The usual complaint of the nurse is that advice upon the nursing of these cases is vague and consists largely of don'ts. But then in the nursing of all patients we may learn much when we know the usual pitfalls that we should try to avoid. Through stepping carefully between one pitfall and the next we generally find that there is a firm path for us to follow, if we only look for it, and our chief guiding light must always be to gain the most thorough understanding that is within our power of the causes and course of any disease we may happen to have in our care. Until this is in our grasp we cannot intelligently nurse any patient, except through luck rather than by judgment. The nurse needs to understand the causes of the characteristic symptoms of pneumonia, for instance, before she can nurse her patient through the onset and crisis, and without knowledge of the course of enteric she would find mere instructions for the care of her patient very complicated to follow. She might be annoyed at the frequent relapses of one suffering from malaria if she did not know the cause of the recurrent pyrexia, and consider the frown and cry of pain from the possessor of a fractured femur *fussy*, when, whilst making the bed, she continually jerked the fracture-boards supporting the uniting fragments of bone, unless her imagination could represent to her the agony she was causing.

It is by no means unusual to find *nervous diseases* put together into one large group without any clear differentiation. Patients will be said to be suffering from nervous debility, hysteria, or neurasthenia without apparent realisation that these terms are not synonymous. This, however, is not the case. We might as well put *infectious diseases* also into one large indeterminate group, without making any distinction between measles, chicken-pox, typhoid, scarlet-fever, tuberculosis, and syphilis. Science has taught the nurse that although all these morbid conditions might be regarded by the layman as having something in common, in so far that they are all *catching* complaints, yet each has a separate character and requires different treatment.

The most common of these terms, *hysteria*, is familiar to everyone, and the adjective *hysterical* is a frequent epithet of opprobrium to designate any member of the female sex who is over-emotional or impulsive. Unfortunately it has become connected in our minds with weakness and the simulation of morbid conditions, which has prejudiced us against nursing the patients suffering from the disorder with the sympathy and understanding we should give to another form of illness, in which the symptoms arose from microbic invasion rather than a disturbance of the mind or the emotions.

In general, a case of neurosis usually conjures up in the

mind of the nurse that of the hysteric, and she also usually regards it with disfavour, since she considers these cases both long and tedious. It is true that often she can make little headway with them, because she does not understand or like them; unless the nurse in question believes she has a special *flair* for this type of work, in which instance they will be exceptionally popular with her.

Let us first consider the various forms of hysteria with which the nurse most often comes in contact, for there are several. If she remains eager for further details concerning such cases she may also refer to the volumes mentioned in the list at the end of this chapter, should her interest or curiosity not have been appeased before. A study of hysteria is essential for another reason besides. Although she may not have been called in to nurse her patient for this disease in the first place, hysterical symptoms will often form a most hindering concomitant of any other trouble, or may appear during convalescence.

We are fond of referring to the "hysterical disposition," and group under this term all who suffer from a mild, chronic form of the disease. They are easily excited, transported with joy, as well as being victims of despair, exaggeratedly optimistic or pessimistic, changing from one extreme to another with lightning rapidity, and *upset* without adequate cause that we know. The best definition is that these persons "suffer from disproportionate emotions," because the known cause, which is believed to stimulate this emotional reaction, seems to the onlooker out of proportion to the stimulus. And yet, if we recollect the brief summary of Freud's discoveries given in the previous chapter, it has been found that the real cause of the emotional outburst is often forgotten, and the present-day cause only one that faintly resembles it, but which, nevertheless, has served to call up this echo from the past.

It is also frequently stated that the hysteric is lacking in control of the Self and the emotions, which is a far from accurate state of affairs in many cases. The hysteric is frequently a person who has at last broken down from exhaustion after a most heroic struggle to maintain self-control that has been unrecognised by friends and relations, sometimes also by the patient. The tension after being too long maintained has given way, or the symptom has been established to retain self-control, being now symbolised in the body, as a defence against the mind surrendering to a lowered moral standard. These cases will require further explanation with greater details later, at present one wishes to give a preliminary outline of the chief causes of hysteria. It is true, however, to say that in a number of cases the patients' emotions may not be under the control of the conscious mind. But psychology, and especially that application of the science which has come to the assistance of medicine, explains many of the most baffling phenomena of human behaviour by the representation that part of our mind has a content and function of which we are not generally aware, and over which our conscious mind has little or no control. This is the *unconscious mind* in which our childish impulses and desires continue to survive. They are for the most part ego-centric, and show but little capacity to be influenced by later experiences, but perpetually seek gratification for the eternal wishes of childhood, often striving to gain through the medium of illness some advantages or an effect that could not be achieved otherwise.

Through the hysterical symptom the patient often seeks to escape from some circumstance, to gain a coveted privilege, or to exert power over persons and things otherwise not possible to control. We should also not forget the repetitive factor in the hysteric symptom, which causes a tendency to repeat old illnesses experienced many years before at the same time of year, or when any circumstance connected with the original occurrence should recur. In his first work upon Hysteria, written in conjunction with Breuer, Freud points out that "hysterical patients suffer principally from reminiscences." (Collected Works, Vol. I. In the original, "Der Hysterische leide grossenteils an Reminiszenzen," *Studien über Hysterie*, von Dr. Josef Breuer und Professor Dr. Sigmund Freud in Wien, Franz Deutike, 1st edition, 1895.)

This mild, constant form of the disease will be found in many persons showing an acute stage also. Hysterical attacks may take place with great suddenness, and often of a severity which causes them to be confused with epilepsy, or fears of different kinds will cause the sufferer to curtail his or her life activities to a very great extent.

In these cases of *Anxiety Hysteria*, as they are called, we find some fear taking almost complete possession of the patient; sometimes it will be linked to a probable occurrence, at others the possibility of meeting with the calamity that is the object of the anxiety is remote. Nevertheless, whenever this anxiety is brought to the mind, the proximity of a cat, a thunderstorm, the possibility of contracting a disease, an accident happening to another person, all the symptoms of extreme terror or anxiety are experienced, trembling, palpitations, breathlessness, sweating, faintness, and maybe tears or laughter. These fears have been given the name of phobias, and some, no doubt, are familiar enough to us from experience: *claustrophobia*, fear of being shut in an enclosed space, of being buried alive; *agoraphobia*, dread of open spaces; *nosophobia*, dread of disease; also fear of the dark or water, death or poverty, as well as of some animals, reptiles, birds, or insects.

In many cases it is difficult to distinguish between *Anxiety Hysteria* and *Anxiety Neurosis*, in both of which nervous anxiety and extreme apprehension with the accompanying symptoms that have been described take a leading part. In his masterly book, *Survey, Development of the Psycho-analytical Theory of the Psychoses, 1894–1926*, Dr. John Rickman points out this difficulty in distinguishing these two forms of neurotic trouble, and remarks that one of the most practical points of difference is that in the former the reactions of the patient are on the whole of a more infantile type.

We shall often find that the actual fear is disguised by a displacement upon a *cover-fear*, which acts as a defence, since the anxiety connected with the substitute fear entirely prevents the patient putting him or herself in such a situation that the real fear could be encountered. Thus a patient known to the writer was afraid to go out alone, and was only happy in company with another older person, saying that she felt so lonely. Upon investigation, however, it appeared that it was not really loneliness that appalled her, but she was really afraid of doing something wrong, of stealing something out of a shop, or the like; perhaps being lost, if there was no one there to tell her what she ought and ought not to do. Therefore, if she never went out alone, she would never run this risk of doing something wrong, because the other person would look after her, and would be to blame if she did anything for which she might afterwards get into trouble. In this way she also avoided taking over an adult responsibility for her own actions, and treated the other person who accompanied her as an external conscience.

These cover-fears will frequently take a form which makes it quite impossible for the patient to continue to carry through the daily routine of life. For instance, a cover-fear or defence may take this form: A housewife may develop anxiety about the management of her house, and become afraid of the servants or the cook, so that she dare not go into the kitchen to give her orders, or to see her maids about it at all. What really is at the bottom of this fear would be impossible to guess without spending time and trouble in so doing, but for the time being let us see what will be the immediate consequences of the fear. She takes to her bed, she is ill, therefore she cannot attend to her housekeeping. A professional nurse comes to look after her, and the strange symptoms of *malaise* which are baffling at first. When her condition does not improve, a housekeeper arrives upon the scene also, who takes the complete burden of the household from off her shoulders, and so the worries of the housekeeping and what this means to the patient leave her untouched, because she has placed a defence of fear between herself and the real anxiety.

How could this situation affect a man in his work? and what type of man would be likely to suffer from this kind of nervous trouble? We should probably find one who was not physically very strong, reticent, rather inefficient and work-shy, whose business may be getting more than he can manage properly through prosperity or mismanagement. He first develops a fear of travelling by train, by which he goes to business daily, and it is suggested that he should motor up to town instead. He then finds a fresh difficulty presents itself, he becomes afraid of driving himself through the traffic, and then of any kind of conveyance in case other vehicles may run into him. He therefore stays at home and tries for a time to conduct his affairs over the telephone. But he then feels that the use of the 'phone is dangerous, and in that way one may contract disease, so either his wife has to do it for him or his managing man is obliged to come to him. He then will really bear the brunt of the work at the office, and the blame when things are not attended to when they should have been.

We may see that on the surface the fear may seem remote or even ridiculous to those looking on, but the anxiety shown by the patient under these circumstances causes him or her an intensity of emotion which is by no means simulated. It is, nevertheless, compatible with the real fear that underlies the defence, although it is often too alarming to be acknowledged or even thought about, therefore the other has been substituted in order that it may never come into conscious thought. What some of these underlying fears may be we will discuss later.

Hysteria, however, does not always show itself in this familiar form. It has been called the *Mocking-Bird of Disease,* and medical science has now discovered that the symptoms of many other diseases are found reproduced most faithfully by means of hysteria, which are often most difficult to differentiate from the actual disease itself. The reasons why these should have been adopted will be given in due course, because they have not come into existence through chance.

Another important group of psycho-neuroses that are included among the hysterias are those which take some physical form, among which must be placed in the first rank the hysterical contractures and paralyses. These are called *Conversion Hysteria.* In these cases there is no organic nerve or muscle degeneration to account for the loss of function in the limb, they represent *an idea* in the mind of the patient which is being expressed in a bodily form, and thus misleads the patient as well as in many cases also those who are trying to treat the illness. For this reason, that the symptom obtains something, or avoids something, that is necessary to the comfort or peace of mind of the patient, we often find that these people seem to bear their sufferings with wonderful patience, so much so in fact that it will frequently be the subject of remark. They are patient, however, because of the existence at the same time of some curious advantage that could not be achieved otherwise.

Conversion Hysteria is the name generally given to

symptoms that affect the limbs or external muscles of the body. Similar hysterical changes of function may also affect the lungs and other internal organs, in which case they will be spoken of as *Hypochondria or Fixation Hysteria.*

Traumatic Hysteria usually arises immediately following some accident. It is generally of short duration, unless special circumstances prolong its course, and it may then become permanent. This is a complication that frequently arises should the severity of the results of the accident affect the question of compensation; in which case it is not difficult to see the relation between the persistence of the trouble and the direct gain that is derived through the disability.

Having now given a brief survey of the various types of hysteria, let us now deal with them in greater detail, and examine side by side with the symptoms and what they represent the usual nursing methods that are advised, and discover to what extent they oppose or fulfil the unconscious wishes of the patient who is being nursed, and the nurse who carries them out.

Usually the nurse is not professionally concerned with the milder forms of Hysteria as such, although they will constantly provide considerable difficulties when engaged in nursing a patient who is suffering from another disease, or in whom minor or latent hysterical symptoms have been increased or awakened by an operation. Commonly, however, our experience will be that during the acute stages of a physical illness symptoms arising from the mind are in abeyance, because the unconscious wishes are already gaining sufficient gratification in this way, but when the acute stage is passed, or convalescence is reached, the hysteria begins to show itself with full vigour.

Roots of the Common Hysteric Symptoms

Let us now begin an investigation of some of those wishes of childhood which find a more ready gratification in sickness than in health, for this leads us to understand the nurse's position in the triangular situation of disease.

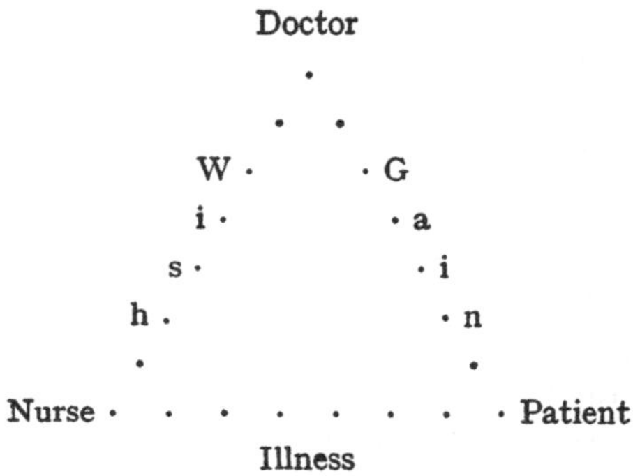

This important triangle may be found with any apex uppermost, and with the names attached to any of the sides changing places or becoming themselves altered; yet the whole idea within the patient's mind is maintained by them until some definite alteration in the imagination devises a different grouping that will transform the figure to conform to a new idea, to represent a different method of gaining the old wish in a more satisfactory guise.

What are the most important wishes of our infancy and childhood that the unconscious mind is always striving to satisfy, often to its disadvantage, or in ways that do not really gain their end, because it is so slow to profit by the actual experience of reality? The wishes that come to the fore throughout our lives, and are especially prominent in hysteria, are, to be the beloved and only child, or, if others must be recognised within the family circle, then to be the *preferred* child, who receives constant and clear proofs of this position of pre-eminence. Freud has pointed out in one of his most recent works concerning the ætiology of neurosis that fear is first aroused by the child's *helplessness* when it realises the absence of the mother. To the child, the mother's absence is equivalent to being altogether abandoned by her. It awakes in the child emotions, to which an adult would attach the realisation that this person who was formerly always affectionately present had now partially, if not entirely, withdrawn her love, and hence her company. (*Hemmung, Symptom und Angst*, Sigmund Freud, Int. Psychoanalytischer Verlag. Wien.)

The chief neurotic or hysteric striving is to gain love at all costs, and to be assured of the protection and the presence of the loved person, upon whom the patient feels as dependent as the infant. Should reality present the stern truth, that these are not so constantly available as before, some process may be set in motion to reverse this state of affairs in reality, or, failing this, in phantasy. Sometimes the truth will be resolutely denied by the mind. In very early years a child may learn thus to juggle with the acceptance of an unwished-for reality; it may likewise be forgotten, reversed, or remembered quite incorrectly by the child, in order to preserve a faked memory that is more in accordance with its wishes.

We often find that an infant who wakes to find itself alone will cry violently to recall the mother. Should this method fail to produce the desired effect, it may scream with increasing emotion of fear until a momentary lapse of consciousness take place, or it sometimes suddenly drops asleep. This stage of unconsciousness will occur at the climax of the fear, beyond which the child cannot find adequate discharge for the terror that has been aroused by the discovery of the missing mother, and serves as a substitute way of escape from the horror of the situation which cannot be resolved otherwise. It will be found to take place not only in infants, but in some persons of all ages when confronted by overwhelming terror (anxiety). The same situation may be seen in the hysterical attack that includes a period of unconsciousness, for which reason this form may often be mistaken for epilepsy: *petit mal* when the unconsciousness is but momentary, but *grand mal* should we have a longer duration, although in character the attacks differ considerably.

It is interesting to observe exactly when these epileptiform attacks occur, what circumstance has immediately preceded them. It is through these differences of causation and also their character, what special symptoms take place while the attack is in progress, which allow of differentiation between the acute hysterical attack and true epilepsy. In some cases not only is the tension of the moment relieved by the loss of consciousness, but extended subsequent amnesia remains, whereby the patient has no recollection afterwards of what has happened nor of the events which led to the attack.

So in early childhood the attempt to sweep from the mind the terrible possibility of being forsaken by the mother seeks to obliterate both the memory as well as the fear, because to retain them would involve the recognition that a similar menace to one's peace of mind, or even to life itself, might occur at any time, since "what has happened once may happen again," as well as the corollary, "if I have ever been deserted once, I can never have been truly loved."

This yearning for love, attention, and protection will be repeated throughout the child's life in countless forms, so that any diminution of attention will recall the old fear, which, although slumbering, is not eradicated, and we shall see the child falling back upon the same tactics to obtain the old wish. The arrival of a new baby in the family is a frequent cause for jealousy, and emotions are aroused which demand some comparable discharge as well as a form of compensation. We may watch similar effects of jealousy in the reactions of hysterical patients in our experiences of ward nursing.

To be loved, to be certain of love, or to be constantly

reassured of it by adequate proofs, are what some children need. The more sensitive or desirous of love the child may be constitutionally, the more strongly it will react to any situation in which its love requirement seems to fall short of expectation. Another dangerous point in the life of the child is going to school, or being introduced for the first time to any sort of training, whether this be carried out by the mother or a stranger. To some children, for the parents to disapprove or to suggest another way of behaviour is an equivalent to a proof of waning affection. The child reasons thus, that if the mother perfectly loved her child, then everything that the child did would be perfect in her eyes, and she would not wish for any alteration. Therefore the wish for improvement is taken as an implied injury from which the child recoils. The same idea may occur to the child once more in connection with being sent away to school, that it is a proof of diminished affection, and is never really forgiven.

Now, let us see how these childish wishes and griefs, struggles and refusals to accept reality may affect the nervous welfare of the child, and the part they may play subsequently in the formation of the so-called hysterical disposition and the symptoms of hysteria.

We have all remarked that the most typical symptoms that we associate with hysteria are already present in a great number of children, some of them, indeed, being the normal emotional reactions of the young child, the abnormality becoming apparent only when they appear in the adult instead of the child. It is more natural for a young child to cry when disappointed, hurt, or frightened than for it to assume stoical self-control. The child also is easily excited, shows signs of manifest pleasure at a small treat; acts upon impulse without forethought, and is overwhelmed with grief or shame when those it loves are not pleased or have punished it. All these tendencies we accept from the child as normal behaviour up to a point. As the years pass by we find that experience and increase of fresh stimuli make the child less easily aroused to emotional response, or rather because greater familiarity with the events of life makes an increased stimulus necessary to produce an emotional reaction of pleasure or of pain. We say the child is growing-up, becoming more self-controlled or blasé, which we prefer: the latter if we should be disappointed that something we have prepared has not called up a response to satisfy us, and self-controlled should the child meet with our approbation.

The same childlike reactions will be seen in the hysteric patient of some types. Faced with occurrences of a certain kind, we find that he or she has either remained emotionally a child or on account of some shock or unbearable situation has made a regression to this stage of life, when difficulties were more easily dealt with, or when life did not present so many, when wishes might be more readily obtained, and when some of the most undesirable situations of adult life never occur at all, and therefore can present no problems.

We say the hysteric constantly seeks love and the proofs of love, wishes for preference and admiration. This is a familiar accusation, and a usual method of dealing with the desire is to find a nurse who can deal firmly with the delinquent, for such is often the opinion held of such a patient. In this way an old situation will frequently be repeated of engaging a strict nursery nurse or governess for a spoilt little boy or girl, who was handed over to a disciplinarian when the mother could manage the child herself no longer.

In point of fact the adult hysteric was frequently the spoilt and charming child of the family, who in the past ruled the family with an iron rod of tears or tantrums, or got her whims and wishes gratified by means of adroitly coaxing some parental authority to let her have her own way, usually the parent of the opposite sex. The little girl wheedled her father, the boy got round his mother, or sulked until she let him do as he wished for the sake of peace and quietness. Something has gone astray in the life of the hysteric, the over-emotional person, with the constitutional need for more love, or a more demonstrative love than others, and has prevented growing-up out of this early need to be loved in this way as a reassurance that he or she will not be deserted and be left alone, unprotected and unloved—helpless. In order to get or maintain love, the symptom takes place to win it by tears, flattery, and cajolery, or even by tempers and bullying.

In the symptoms and the way they are used we meet the eternal triangle of the nursery once again, reproduced in the sick-room as soon as the doctor calls in the nurse. Medical men are often, unconsciously if not consciously, flattered by the appeal for their help from the female hysteric, especially if she be young and attractive. But the hysterical woman, when she gains a certain amount of attention and protectiveness, becomes increasingly insistent in her demands. For this reason she will change in the eyes of the doctor from being a pleasant, obedient patient into a bore, and the nurse will be called in to deal with her. We should likewise recollect that the male hysteric, who is usually endowed with a large share of those tendencies which we generally associate with a woman, and who probably may have wished to have been a girl at some period of his life, for these reasons may be equally prone to want to seek the help and protection of a substitute father in the person of the medical man, although he will not be aware of this motive, or very rarely.

The stage is now set. We have a substitute father in the doctor, a mother in the nurse, and a child between them, hungering for love and attention, in the patient, who reaches this goal through the illness, which could scarcely be so well obtained in any other setting. The danger of many forms of nerve cure is that they play into the hands of the patient, who thus wants to go back to happy, irresponsible childhood, and lead to the unfortunate result that recovery is so slow, and may even then not be permanent. In this case the patient frequently shows an inclination to relapse when life once more becomes monotonous or difficult, and the sheltered atmosphere of the rest-cure, where one is the centre of much attention, offers a vastly preferable alternative.

What, then, can the nurse do from her triangle-corner (see p. 70) to free the patient from this malady of wishes gone astray? She must hope that the doctor is using some form of psycho-therapy, which will in time bring the facts of the case into the consciousness of the patient, because, certainly at the beginning, the patient does not realise the cause of the illness, but believes it has nothing to do with him or herself, but that it is an affliction from Providence or some external source, as much as, let us say, the measles.

To show the patient that the nurse believes the illness to have been caused by the mind, or the wish to escape from something in life, would give the patient the idea that the nurse felt she was pretending, which would in all probability lead to an exacerbation of the symptoms at once, to prove that they were genuine. Neither must the nurse fall into the trap of the *Transference Situation*, by which the patient transfers all old childish feelings felt for another upon the nurse, as we have already described above, calling the sick-room the repetition of the nursery triangle.

It is equally dangerous to be a provider of too much gratification for the old childish wishes, since in this way the illness may tend to become permanent, in order to retain this loving protector always. But sometimes the child in the hysterical adult wants the stern mother, who will supply the deficiency of her own will-power, and be willing to act as an external conscience, as in the case we have already quoted. It is by no means rare to find the wealthy hysteric permanently afflicted with some mild form of bodily illness, which is just sufficient to need the attention of a resident nurse. This situation may then fulfil so many of the patient's unconscious wishes, should the nurse settle down into playing the part required of her in the illness, that cure or recovery will most probably never take place, because it would mean separation from the protector, and thus repetition of the greatest trauma of childhood.

We have said that the nurse must not fall into the trap of the Transference Situation. What is this, and why should it be so sedulously avoided? This name, Transference Situation, has been given to a psychological mechanism, by which one person transfers to another feelings or thoughts that originally belonged to someone known in the past, whom this new figure resembles in some way. Thus the nurse called in to attend to a hysteric patient will, because of her care and attention, remind her patient of all the love and help derived by the child from some dearly loved mother or nurse, who bestowed similar ministrations upon her when a helpless little child. Starting with this one point of resemblance, others will follow, and we will frequently hear patients say that the nurse is like somebody, but they cannot remember who it is, or that she reminds them of some person they knew long ago, sometimes recognising the original, but occasionally not being able to do so at all.

Other supplementary difficulties may arise from the Transference and offer complications for the nurse in charge of the case. Because of the partial resemblance, the unconscious mind of the patient tries to put this *imago* or parent substitute entirely in the place of the original figure, and expect identical behaviour from her, so that just as much love and care will be expected as from the mother of old.

Or, should the parent have been dominating, and controlled the child by threats and fear, an equal amount of rigid discipline will be expected from the nurse, the patient acting in such a way as to make it almost compulsory for the nurse to respond according to the patient's wishes, and so taking an active part in this repertory play from childhood. This is the trap set for the nurse and baited by the patient's wishes, shown in her behaviour.

Why should it be so necessary to warn the nurse to avoid it? Is she not able to see it for herself? Why should she be expected to walk into it so readily? For several reasons, but mainly because she too has an unconscious mind, from which her unfulfilled infantile wishes are likewise seeking gratification, which, unless she is both forewarned and forearmed, go out to welcome those of her patient. What these may be, let us now investigate farther.

The teaching of modern psychology shows us that it is not by chance alone or external opportunities that we are constrained to choose one profession or another. Wishes and events of her own childhood usually lead the nurse to devote her time to the help or charge of sick folk, especially in these days when so many more generally attractive professions are open to the girl than used to be in the past. We cannot follow here, in detail, all the several contributory streams which may have influenced her choice, but may outline very briefly two main groups: those persons whose unconscious wish was to help the poor sick folk who would love her in return, i.e. the tender-hearted nurse, who may be inclined to be almost too sympathetic and sentimental, because in her unconscious mind she sees in them herself, or someone who is or was dear to her, whom she wants to feel dependent upon her loving care. This gentle nurse is usually a Mother Identification. (Note.—By Identification we mean the imitation of another by the self; imaging ourselves in the part of another, and acting as they did, or would, if the object of the identification is an abstract ideal or traditional figure.) Whereas the other group is motivated by the wish for power of some kind, the dominance of the healthy person over the sick, the skilled over the unskilled, the strong over the weak in many symbolic ways, that often proves to be an identification with the father, who was the chief power in the family.

Both these types of nurse will be attracted by psychogenic cases and both may through their own individual methods be successful, provided they come in contact with the right sort of patient, with whose wishes their own kind of personality fits in. Yet, unless these nurses are very careful, and know something of their patients' desires, they will probably before long be dancing to the piping of the patient, rather than calling the tune of the recovery themselves, because the susceptible unconscious mind of the patient has appealed to them for the discharge of the particular wish that is seeking gratification. Love and tender solicitude is coaxed willingly enough out of these gentle nurses, who really long to have a helpless being clinging devotedly to them, although they may tell others that they hate it.

This particular appeal for affection merely bores the stern disciplinarian, and the pull-yourself-together type of nurse with the strong personality, whose unconscious wish for power will be played upon the patient, who as a child was brought up by some dominating mother or nurse, and found by experience that the greatest amount of notice could be gained through being naughty or tiresome, in which case a scolding or perhaps a punishment, because welcomed in the same way as other children yearn for a caress—those being the only possible marks of attention obtainable from authority.

If this relationship between nurse and patient gives such profound gratification to the wishes of both, we may well ask, Why should it be regarded as a trap, about which the nurse must be forewarned and forearmed? Can it then be such a grave danger, and why? If the patient is suffering from hysteria because of a deficiency of love and attention, surely the best means of cure is to provide for the lack. This is true up to a certain point, but beyond this there are certain dangers that must be explained more fully. Many medical treatments consist in equalisation of deficiency through diet, administration of glandular extracts, and so forth. But they cannot be given *ad libitum*, without the exercise of medical control to watch for signs of intolerance, and the patient's idiosyncrasies to this particular substance. Further, we know that some drugs provide a craving for them in ever increasingly large doses, so that their effect may be maintained, and accordingly the physician takes this into his most careful consideration before he prescribes them, lest the last state of the patient be worse than the first.

This might well be the condition brought about in the hysteric patient by the nurse, should the unconscious wishes of both coincide, so that they gave one another constant gratification. The illness would become chronic because an ideal state had been achieved, and the nurse would become established for life as a resident loving protector or a martinet. A fresh neurotic state would have been evolved in exchange for the old one, including two persons, and no cure nor freedom for either could be accomplished until the alliance were resolved. This, of course, might happen in the case of the mutual demands becoming unbearably exacting, until some limit were reached beyond which one of the two would not go. Some wish would be denied, the disappointed person would then feel mortally wounded, and break off the former arrangement. Then the old game might possibly begin anew with someone else, unless the patient, tired for the time being of a surfeit of tenderness, turned to find fresh interests outside the sphere of illness, and appeared temporarily cured by the liberation from the love-object upon which she had become too dependent.

The cure of hysteria cannot be brought about solely by gratifying the craving for love and attention that is the fulfilment of infantile wishes. This is necessary, but it must be carried out by the nurse, who knows as thoroughly what she is about in nursing her patient with this treatment as when she is administering dangerous drugs, serums, or extracts, the effects and after-effects of which it is necessary to watch with the keenest attention. She must know the properties of her own psychology, and what results its components are likely to have upon her patient, so that she can go on or hold back, as in the case of other complicated medical treatment she might be left to carry out, reporting progress at intervals to the doctor in charge of the case. She must, in order to be able to do this, be thoroughly conversant with the origins and course of the disease in general, and observe carefully so that she may gain fresh knowledge through experience of each particular case.

If she holds fast to the conception of hysteria as a disorder of the emotions or the imagination, and does not confound this form of words with the idea that could be derived from changing them round into an *emotional or imaginary trouble*, she will find her work easier. She will discover, when she comes to understand the causes underlying many of the forms of hysteria, that these patients are suffering from a trouble they have fought against for years, which has gradually worn down their resistance against realising a very painful truth, and the illness is their last defence. In such cases it is not conceivable we should scold them out of it, nor laugh them out of it. It cannot be lightly forgotten nor side-tracked by inducing the patient to "think of something more cheerful, or to take up a new kind of fancy needlework." We may think that the ideas of the patients are fantastic and ridiculous, but they are real horrors to them, and their diseased ideas require as much respect and help as the morbid new growths that readily call forth our sympathy in the patient who is suffering from cancer.

The essential factor in the cure of hysteria is the recognition by the patient of the true state of affairs that the symptom represents; and in some cases it has found "that single hysterical symptoms would immediately vanish without recurrence, when it was possible to bring to remembrance all the circumstances with vividness, together with the original affect, particularly if and when the patient described the event in the fullest possible way, and discharged this affect in words. Memories brought up without affect are usually of little therapeutic service." (*Studien über Hysterie*, Dr. Josef Breuer und Professor Dr. Sigmund Freud.) The patient suffers, we are told, from the emotions stored up from long-forgotten memories, that must be restored before they can be released. It is not the nurse's job to perform the mental operation, but to tend and observe the patient meanwhile, and supply, as her valuable contribution to the patient's recovery—herself.

These are some of the main outlines of the difficulties of nursing the hysteric patient, others will be referred to when we come to consider some of the other types of the disorder in further detail. It is easy to recognise the repetition of childhood and its ways in the behaviour of the hysteric patient, whether a man, woman, or even still in childhood, because these symptoms may already appear with severity at an early age, and often require the services of the nurse. Those who have a genuine understanding and sympathy with the ways and thought-processes of children make the best nurses for neurotic cases, but they should at the same time keep steadily before their eyes this ideal, that the pseudo-child needs to grow up again as swiftly and surely as possible.

We see the child's behaviour repeated once again in the patient's reactions to strangers. Frequently the interest of having a new personality to explore will occupy the sick person's attention for days, and careful trial of many experiments will be made to ascertain the full range of the nurse's behaviour under various circumstances. Novelty plays an important part in the illness of the hysteric patient, but sometimes we will find a definite fear or dislike of a stranger, who may offer a rival to the interest that attaches to themselves. Their jealousy is another conspicuous factor in the disorder, and it is always worth while to notice very carefully of whom and when this feeling shows itself, because some situation which formerly resembled this occasion was probably an important element in the development of the trouble. Ward or institutional nursing naturally offers more opportunities for the exhibition of jealousy on the part of patients than when they are being nursed privately or in a nursing-home. Yet every environment presents sooner or later a situation which will provoke jealousy, even the visit of the doctor or the nurse's off-duty time.

There is another notable psychological phenomenon which arises in human beings that we find playing an extremely prominent part among the symptoms of those who are suffering from conversion hysteria especially. This is what is known as *Identification*, which means the imitation of another, one aspect of which has already been described. It may frequently be the determining cause of adoption of one particular symptom. Thus a woman may always have a bad attack of asthma about the anniversary of the death of her father, who died of this complaint many years before; or a man visits every hospital in London to seek reassurance that he has not got a cerebral tumour, which disease, we hear later, was the cause of his mother's death. We visit a friend who has recently been operated upon for acute appendicitis, and come home feeling all the symptoms she has described so vividly. It may also account for patients in a ward adding the symptoms of others to their own. But it will and can also work beneficially, because any personal characteristic may thus be imitated as well as a symptom of illness. This is how a patient's capacity for ready identification concerns the nurse in the process of recovery. The patient, who likes her, will quickly pick up, not only any little mannerism she may happen to possess just as her technical or professional vocabulary may be imitated, but is also capable of co-opting her normal attitude to life, to responsibility, and her possession of mental balance or physical health, if, indeed, they are there to copy. For this reason, that the patient has to grow up again, we need our nurses in charge of psychological patients to be all that one could wish from the standpoint of nervous balance, with a normal attitude towards life and its responsibilities, and possessing more than the average share of attractiveness and good health.

The child originally grows up through this same process of imitating first one person and then another who has been attractive and therefore beloved. We must take this mechanism of Identification into serious consideration in the nursing of our neurotic patients, because it assumes the first position, whether we will or no, among curative functions, or it may prove a serious handicap towards recovery, should the identifications with the nurse be more of a hindrance than a help, because the new symptoms or acquired characteristics are hard to eradicate once they have become established.

The phenomenon, of course, is closely allied to the effects of *Suggestion*, and, in fact, it is actually a manifestation of the result of unconscious suggestion radiated from the personality of the nurse, and adopted by the suggestibility of the patient. We are familiar enough with the idea of using conscious suggestion upon these cases, and the hysteric is supposed to be particularly accessible to this form of therapy, but it requires very careful handling, and is useless or even dangerous when applied clumsily and without expert knowledge. Equal harm may also be done by *inadvertent* suggestion, through the unconsidered remarks of a nurse being acted upon by a patient, which were not meant to serve as suggestions at all. It should also be remembered that many people we meet are what is called *contra-suggestible*, which means that they always take the opposite course to that which has been suggested to them by another person.

We have mentioned that the nurse should make herself conversant as far as possible with the causes of hysteria upon broad outlines, and then fill in details from subsequent observation of her patients. The causes of some of the more usual manifestations of hysterical indisposition have been briefly touched upon already, and it may be as well to add a few explanations of some of the underlying foundations of more specific symptoms that occur in hysteria. It has been pointed out that a symptom may have been borrowed from another person with whom the patient has identified, usually because this other was tenderly loved, or who through the illness gained some advantage the imitator would gladly share. The similarity of the symptom will certainly be recognised by the patient, who may think it strange that it should have made a second appearance in the family, but usually attributes this to heredity, thus believing it to be unavoidable on this account. The idea that it has been caused by a mental process without a physical causation never reaches consciousness, still less the idea that there is a stronger dynamic yet, which is the wish to gain what this prototype is supposed to have derived from the malady. It is a difficult and lengthy process to introduce this new attitude to the conscious mind of the patient, and so bring about the cure, and it should without doubt only be attempted by an expert practitioner of psychotherapy.

The secondary gain of the illness is one of the greatest obstacles to be encountered in the cure of psychological disease. It was realised first in the conditions known as *Traumatic Hysteria* or *Neurosis*, where the trouble had been apparently caused by an accident, or, as in some cases of shell-shock, by an accident or injury preceded by a long period of overstrain. When distinct financial gain is to be acquired from injury to the body or to general health, which will cease altogether, or be decreased through recovery, it is difficult to cure the patient, although he or she may believe this desire for recovery to be strong. This same factor will also present incalculable difficulties when return to health means that the patient once more becomes *just an ordinary person*, robbed of the certain glamour which illness lends, one who has not much social or intellectual interest to offer to attract friends, who is not sufficiently well off to provide much diversion or amusement in life, and for whom the daily round of a humdrum existence is all the future has to offer. To be ill, to be interesting, to be able to command a certain amount of attention from doctors, nurses, relations, and friends, perhaps also from fellow-patients as well, seems a far preferable thing, and so one interesting or startling symptom appears after another to keep up the interest and prevent it flagging from monotony.

The hysterical symptom may frequently represent an abstract idea in the patient's mind, one which would not be allowed a place in the conscious thoughts of this same person, who never for an instant recognises the meaning of this somatic language. This is the form of hysteria to which we have referred particularly when mentioning that an hysterical symptom, usually of a physical nature, is established unconsciously to maintain emotional self-control. Thus nausea or hysterical vomiting will often mean that the patient is mentally *sick about something*, such as his or her own treatment by another, or may use the symbol to express moral disapproval. The patient who suffers from *globus hystericus*, the feeling that it is impossible to swallow, may really be giving a physical form to the corresponding thought, "I cannot swallow that," or "such behaviour sticks in my throat." What this behaviour is, or what proves so unpalatable, must be discovered before the person may be relieved of the distressing symptom. We also often find that severe headache of the migraine type will arise from suppressed anger, or will be due to a feeling of resentment which the sufferer was unable to express directly and verbally. Or the headache will prevent visits to relations.

Closely allied to this particular mechanism as an originator of hysterical symptoms will be found the causative factors of *psychological blindness and deafness*, which may often occur in adults as well as in children. The patient develops this symptom suddenly or by degrees, and after examination no physical root can be traced to account for its onset. After a long and arduous psycho-analytic investigation the cause will generally be found to be of this nature. There is someone or something that the patient wishes to sweep out of existence, to remain blind to or deaf to. The person or thing cannot be abolished, so the only alternative is that of the child, who, wishing to escape from the ugly faces seen on the wallpaper by a flickering nightlight, shuts its eyes and so accomplishes it as though by magic. The person or thing disappears. The same psychological process remains valid in some cases without shutting the eyes: "Eyes have they, but they see not, ears have they, but they hear not." The child who becomes psychologically deaf often does so to remain oblivious of the cries of a little rival, or the loving words of the mother who comforts another.

The mind can in this way abolish actual sounds that we

do not wish to hear, but with equal facility it can create others that might be desired, or invent angry, incriminating voices in hallucinations, which are generally the result of other conditions in nervous disorder, to be explained in the following chapter. One is the reverse of the other, both equally the result of a wish and arising within the unconscious mind of the patient.

In the preliminary outline of the different forms of Hysteria given at the commencement of this chapter, Conversion Hysteria was mentioned, together with the closely allied *Hypochondria* or *Fixation Hysteria*, which will show among its chief symptoms those connected with the gastro-intestinal tract or the respiratory organs. These conditions are often a cause of difficulty to the nurse, worrying and interesting many because so little information is to be found about them in nursing textbooks. The nurse may gather that there is no adequate somatic cause to be found for the paralysis or contracture, but she seldom gleans an alternative suggestion as to how it has been derived. In the past she noticed that these cases were treated by electric battery, massage, perhaps by hydrotherapy, occasionally hypnotism—although in England this would generally be *sub rosa*—some were cured by these means, some were not. They would be moved on from the hospital where she was working, and she lost sight of them. The same would happen also in private work, unless she settled down as a faithful attendant for the life of her patient. Otherwise she became tired of the monotony and went on to another case, or the institution for which she was working moved her at the end of her allotted time, and so she lost touch with the patient's progress and the subsequent history of the case.

During the war an interesting series of Medical Handbooks were published by the London University Press, including two which dealt with these psychogenic conditions:

one, *The Psycho-neuroses of War*, by G. Roussey and J. L'Hermitte, edited by William Aldren Turner, C.B., M.D.; the other, *Hysteria or Pithiatism*, by J. Babinski and J. Froment, edited by E. Farquhar Buzzard. (See list of books appended to last chapter.) In these one may find a most interesting account of cases and various curative methods used at that time, which comprise electricity and various other rather violent therapeutic measures, in which the authors evidently seemed to repose the utmost confidence. No rules for nursing these patients, however, are given; nor, indeed, are the nurses in charge of them mentioned at all, except in a short paragraph to point out that the sympathy and considerate attention of these persons act as the most powerful suggestion *to make the patients believe they are more seriously afflicted than is the case.*

A useful book on the subject appeared in 1928, published by the American firm, W. B. Saunders Company, entitled *Nervous and Mental Diseases for Nurses*, by Irving J. Sands, M.D., a leading neurologist, in which he certainly offers a considerable amount of information to nurses engaged in the care of serious cases of neurological and mental diseases, generally being nursed in State Hospitals and Institutions. Physical treatment for these conditions seems advised in the place of chief importance, although the author acknowledges that for many cases of sufficient intelligence and education to profit by it, psycho-analysis "offers the best form of therapy. It is the most efficient form, etc." Yet from details appended he seems to have gained experience of results, not at first-hand, but quite remotely. His assistance to nurses is mainly to direct them in the care of the patient's body; although he acknowledges that the disease springs from mechanisms within the mind of the patient, this seems to receive practically no attention unless a doctor is providing psycho-analytic treatment for the intelligent and educated patients. High colonic irrigation, enemata, instructions in the use of the tooth-brush, encouragement to be given to female patients to make use of Beauty Parlours provided for them in the State Institutions, to see that patients take exercise in the fresh air and have a liberal diet seems to include all that the nurse need concern herself with in regard to her patients; then she takes care of her own ethical behaviour, and her whole duty is accomplished, according to this manual for nurses. Yet at first glance it seemed so promising, and also is, so far as it goes; but it stops short of understanding the real questions that concern the nursing of these patients, the influence of the nurse upon her patient, and that of the patient upon the nurse, as well as the many practical problems that await us daily.

The nurse is often in an exceedingly onerous position with regard to these cases. Let us imagine this by no means uncommon situation. A doctor in private practice tells the nurse that there is absolutely nothing physical the matter with a patient who believes she has injured her spine, but at the same time leads the patient to believe that her own conjecture is correct, and advises massage, hoping that the suggestive influence of the treatment will have the desired effect and restore her to health. As it happens the pain continues, because the source—a complexity of feelings aroused by a lifetime of jealousy directed against an elder sister whom the patient imagined threw the chair at her and caused the injury—remains unrelieved. The chair, however, did not touch the patient, but had fallen with a loud crash behind her. The immediate result was that she remained bedridden for a long time, followed by years of impaired health and painful walking, until subsequently relieved by psycho-analysis, which disclosed the true state of affairs.

When the nurse is asked by the patient in this case why the pain in her back is not improved by the massage as the doctor predicted, what can she say, particularly when she has been given a clear statement that it is caused by a mental process, although he has led her patient to keep her belief in a physical one? In these cases the nurse carries out all the treatment prescribed by the medical man for the corresponding physical condition, refers the patient to the doctor himself for a reply to her question, and may truthfully reply that she "cannot say!" which is a protective method between medical etiquette and an inquiring patient. The nurse in such a case may always hope that some day her patient will meet with a medical man who will understand her case and set about its cure, and trust that in the meantime the phenomenon of identification will come to the rescue and play its part in the re-establishment of the patient's health.

Many patients, requiring only a plausible excuse to get well that any treatment gives, respond to it with surprising and gratifying rapidity, and are easily accessible to curative suggestion of all kinds. Massage is of the greatest value to many for this reason, and is rapidly coming into favour as a successful treatment; but to what extent the active principle is really suggestion is an open question. It will also have the effect of redirecting the patient's thoughts regarding this particular part of the body into fresh channels, and perhaps investing the movements with new rhythmical opportunities for pleasure instead of the old associations of pain. Muscle pleasure and muscle pain are important subjects that have as yet not been fully investigated.

Behind bodily pain an idea of *guilt* and an attempt at self-punishment will frequently be hidden; let us remember the result of a product of the Unconscious Mind, which aims at a complex representation in one symptom of some secondary gain in illness, the repetition of some traumatic incident of the past, self-punishment connected with an idea of guilt, and a bid for pity. This over-determination of symptoms as they are called, when they represent so many different factors in combination, offer a fund of interesting material to the nurse in charge of the case, so that anyone with a tendency to scientific research and a genuine interest in the complexity of the human mind as shown by such manifestations cannot truly complain that the nursing of Hysteria is either monotonous or dull.

NOTE TO CHAPTER II

It has been pointed out several times in the course of this chapter that the nurse should have a thorough knowledge of herself, her psychological make-up, and her unconscious tendencies, before she can successfully nurse those troubled with nervous diseases.

How is she to equip herself with this knowledge is a question which will doubtless occur to many readers. The most valuable advice that can be offered to her to solve the difficulty is that in addition to reading such books as will give her the technical information necessary for her work, she herself should also have the experience of a course of psycho-analysis, carried out by a competent, fully-trained psycho-analyst.

This will not only give her a wider knowledge of the subject than can be obtained in other ways, but it will help to resolve her own complexes, which would otherwise place serious obstacles in the way of the understanding of patients' difficulties, or cause her to react in an injurious way to their manifestations of neurosis. In many cases the nursing of nervous diseases awaken the most violent reverberations and guilt in the deeper structures of the nurse's unconscious mind, which disturb her as well as her patient. Through her own analysis, these would be checked to the great benefit of all concerned.

CHAPTER III

NEURASTHENIA AND OBSESSIONAL NEUROSES

NEURASTHENIA

It is now over forty years ago since Van Deusen introduced the name of Neurasthenia to the medical world, and it has become a comprehensive title for many varying kinds of psychogenic disorders not obviously hysterical.

True, Neurasthenia may best be described as a *fatigue disease,* because the most general symptom which appears on the surface is that of nervous exhaustion, popularly known as brain-fag, together with difficulty in concentration of attention. The patient will complain frequently of a sensation of pressure on the head and an irritable spine; gastro-intestinal symptoms are also common, most general amongst which will be found to be constipation and flatulent dyspepsia. The person gradually withdraws his or her interest and attention from outside affairs to centre it entirely upon this condition of ill-health.

When we come to investigate the origins of this primary fatigue neurosis, we arrive at the important question, Do we find this condition most often arising from actual causes of great or prolonged physical and mental strain, such as overwork, extreme anxiety, even the aftermath of illness, or are we confronted with a psychological condition, an adequate cause for which it is difficult to assign?

To answer this question correctly we must leave the easy path of generalisation and examine in detail several possibilities. It is very seldom, when we come to investigate psycho-neuroses, that we find them attributable to one cause alone, such as occurs in the case of those due to germ infection or physical degeneration of tissue. We usually find the neurotic symptom arising as a vehicle of many convergent ideas and allied origins, as well as being the product of various causes. It is only when we have some knowledge of the cause of the trouble, however, that an appropriate remedy or treatment may be determined.

This nervous exhaustion, of which sufferers from neurasthenia complain, may indeed arise after prolonged physical or mental strain, some kinds of physical illness such as influenza, or a constant state of underfeeding. In these cases the cessation of the strain, recovery of normal health after convalescence, and a restoration of nourishing diet will doubtless lead to the recovery of the patient's nervous health. When we find, however, that recuperation of physical and mental energy does not follow with the lapse of time and improvement in the conditions, which were supposed to have been responsible for the lack of health on the part of the patient, it is necessary to look farther for the cause, and therefore an indication of the cure necessary for this form of neurosis.

Let us take first the study of the symptom of *inertia*, which we will often find becoming permanent after a period of overwork or anxiety. What other factors may contribute to its radication? We have already mentioned the importance of the secondary gain of illness, which frequently accounts for the fixation of nervous invalidism. The sick person may, and usually does, command greater consideration and sympathy than those who are inconspicuously healthy, and at the same time is permitted to indulge in idleness and luxury to a greater extent than those who remain in robust health, from whom work and service for others is commonly expected. Illness also carries with it the right to escape from unwanted responsibility, while various other advantages are acquired, including the before-mentioned feeling of justification for self-indulgence and a far-reaching influence over household arrangements and the affairs of friends and relatives. A large amount of reconstruction must necessarily take place in the routine of a household to conform with the needs of an invalid, who usually takes advantage of this necessity to increase it with the help of medical authority, for the doctor will occasionally deliver the dictum that anything which may upset the patient is best avoided. "I must not be worried," or "I must not be upset, it is so bad for my nerves," thus becomes the patient's most valuable weapon of offence and defence. The man or woman who adopts this refuge, then, has the opportunity to refuse utterly to tackle any situation which seems to contain a mere possibility of worry, thus permanently anchoring in a pleasant backwater of life, where no storms may enter, and keeping others in a constant state of threat of increased illness should the wished-for conditions not be complied with.

This condition of continued illness may therefore become the result of an unconscious insurance scheme against a recurrence of the original cause of the trouble, such as may occasionally find expression in such words as these: "Once is enough, you don't catch me doing that again. But then I could not, if I wanted to, my health would never allow it!" or, "I have worked sufficient for a lifetime, somebody else can wait upon me now." An undercurrent of defence of this description will usually be found to be the cause of those forms of nervous illness which have been called *Occupational Neurosis,* to which we will refer with more detail in a later chapter.

Another cause of the consequences of overstrain becoming permanent may be to provide a visible reproach against the person or condition which has caused the breakdown, in conjunction with the wish to gain compensation for the injury that has been already sustained. This motive of unconscious revenge is a difficult state of mind to deal with, because it offers the deepest resistance to becoming conscious, since any yielding of the condition to treatment would be tantamount to admission that the guilt of the other person had not been so grievous after all, nor the effects so injurious. It would be necessary, before recovery could take place, for this patient to discover a still greater advantage in health than in ill-health, or that it was worth while to surrender the hostility against the old enemy to make room for a new and more happy allegiance to some fresh protector, with whom a constructive identification has been made. This condition would probably occur most frequently in conjunction with the transference to doctor or nurse, who is essentially on the side of regaining health. It must appear to these patients worth while to recover for some good reason, or it will not be achieved, and we will be told in a voice of triumph how many doctors have been visited, all of whom were quite powerless to make the least impression upon this lowered vitality and increasing inertia, which suggests that the sick may unconsciously, if not consciously, believe a battle to be won through the maintenance of the disease.

The subject of Guilt plays a remarkable part in both the two forms of nervous trouble that occupy our attention in this chapter—Neurasthenia and Obsessional Neurosis. Prolonged illness of a neurotic origin appearing as neurasthenia may frequently occur after the death of some relative, whom the patient has been nursing for a long time with a devotion which actually did entail great physical and mental strain. When the confidence of the patient has been won, we will often hear of some haunting dread that she has been in some way responsible for the death of this relative, through ignorance or neglect, and in some cases even we become aware of an idea in our patient's mind that she had taken some active step to secure release from the situation that was becoming intolerable. Frequently these self-accusations are entirely unfounded, but they will continue, no matter how often the nurse may explain the impossibility of her present patient being in any way to blame for the fatal termination of the illness.

In such a case the guilt arises from a feeling, which may have been conscious or not, that the death of this relative would be an advantage. We should bear in mind in this connection that an unconscious death-wish, or one which has been contested most strenuously by the patient's moral code, will be more likely to lead to the formation of nervous symptoms than one which is clearly recognised as inevitable, in these cases of an incurable, painful, or prolonged illness of a relation. The second illness, therefore, that has been produced from feelings of guilt concerning the first shows this condition playing the part of a punishment and atonement for neglect or of whatever the patient accuses herself.

A nurse in charge of such a case will find herself appealed to frequently by her patient for reassurance of all kinds, but in some way connected with this fear and guilt. She may also be puzzled by requests for information concerning some form of physical illness before she has been confided in to the extent I have described. Many and detailed inquiries about the nursing of patients suffering from one particular illness, the precautions that should be taken in the administration of drugs or against the spread of infection, may well arouse a nurse's suspicions that some worry of this nature is causing a disturbance in the mind of her patient.

The nurse in such a case will need to reflect that it is not going to be an easy matter to convince her patient of the mistake which she has made in attributing the death of the relative to some want of care or overt act of violence. The inability to believe her innocence is compatible with the force of the unconscious death-wish, and the desire to atone for it by self-punishment through the continuance of the illness or anxiety. We will also find another symptom at work taking an important part in the structure of the Obsessional Neurosis that partakes of the same nature, which is *Doubt*, allied to the Doubting Mania of the psychiatrists.

These persons now afflicted with torturing doubts were in many instances originally embued with a great sense of their own importance and power, for good or evil. They wanted to feel that their wishes were omnipotent, and that their slightest whim would be instantly gratified as soon as it should find expression. Reality, nevertheless, often proved the contrary, but when convenient the patient would still continue to struggle against the evidence of truth and fact, because of this wish to retain belief in a more welcome phantasy. In this way conflict arises concerning wishes and the belief in their own power, and consequently the ability readily to be persuaded that personal guilt has been less than supposed carries with it the corollary that the influence of the wish can also not have been so far-reaching nor so powerful. This is an admission the unconscious mind is loath to make, although in many ways peace of mind might be obtained in the process. Unconscious desires for power or proofs of power will often for this reason maintain their struggle to the disadvantage of the conscious interests of a person suffering from obsessional neurosis or from neurasthenia.

The nurse in charge of the neurasthenic or obsessional patient will therefore often find herself obliged frequently to answer the same question, to reiterate the same reassurance, and find fresh proofs of the innocence of her patient, should such be available, accurate, and ready to hand. After countless repetitions they *may* at last bear permanent fruit, especially should the patient discover that her nurse's word may be relied upon in other ways, and her compliance with the anxious requests for comfort will usually afford relief at the moment. A more permanent effect can hardly be hoped for in the most acute cases of this trouble, from such a superficial palliative for a condition of which it is but one sign, although one that is indicative that the attention of a medical specialist in this form of nervous disease is needed without delay.

For one who is not experienced in nursing obsessional patients this failure to respond to her assurances will often be extremely trying to the nurse's patience, as well as presenting difficulties to her comprehension of the condition before her. Upon the surface it seems incredible that an adult, intelligent enough in other ways, can continue to believe what seems to her to be such utter nonsense, or that a fresh outbreak of the doubt should arise after it had been once or even many times proved to be erroneous and totally without foundation. This usually means that the nurse herself is also not entirely without some wish for omnipotence, and possesses a desire for power that becomes ruffled when her word of authority does not have the required effect. To be able to cure or calm a patient's mind by our words conjures up in our minds the actions of the ancient miracle workers, and arouses the love of magic that slumbers in most of us, particularly in those who devote their lives to the ministration of the sick. We should therefore be on our guard against any clear demonstration of our own importance or consequent impatience, keeping very strictly within the confines of accuracy when we are trying to calm the fears of our patients, because they will usually remember what we have said on previous occasions and be able to refute us with our own words should they not tally.

The confidences of patients are always a grave responsibility for any medical attendant, but become especially onerous to the nurse engaged upon private work of this kind, and connected with them she may find many perplexities. Those who have had opportunity to obtain the confidence of their patients and thus hear details of their lives, which have often been kept secret from their nearest and dearest, are fully conversant with the fact that in the past history of patients suffering from nervous diseases we discover many troubles, disappointments, and abnormalities, connected with what we may call their *love-life*. Freud has been pilloried constantly in the past for his insistence that sexual disturbances have been one of the prime factors in the ætiology of the neuroses. He has also pointed out the morbid effects of undue repression of the sexual instinct, as well as the consequences of the conflict between this instinct and the Ego Impulses at the instance of the Super-Ego, the moral conscience, that is often over-developed to the extent of exerting a crippling limitation to the functions of the Ego, since only by limiting these functions, or a wide series of those which are contingent, can the sexual interest and all that appertains to it be duly brought into subjection.

Those who have come in contact with living persons suffering from these disorders, and who learn their troubles first-hand, will admit the truth of these statements. Sooner or later, when our patients feel they can rely upon our respecting their confidence, they will tell us the true state of affairs, or give us information relative to themselves or others, which will corroborate for us the teaching of Freud. Frequently they will indeed give us these details without recognising their importance, or realising how they are actually causing the symptoms that are proving so distressing or persistent.

Still, once in possession of these important facts, how are we to deal with them? Patients will often tell the nurse things of this kind to appeal to her sympathy and try to get her to take sides, perhaps even to take some action in the matter by making overtures to the other persons concerned. This contingency the nurse will have to deal with in a tactful way, but steadily avoid taking any active part in the affairs of her patient, although when her sympathies have been aroused it may be difficult for her to refrain from so doing. This is another instance when a nurse in charge of the nervous patient requires to watch her own reactions with the utmost care and prevent her own psychological proclivities affecting her treatment of the patient or the friends and relatives.

There is still another side, however, What may we do where our patient is concerned? Sometimes we will be able to point out an obvious connection here and there, but only when it has become so clear through constant repetition that it cannot be missed. However, the mere fact of being able to talk of these worries to somebody who understands the trouble such things may cause, who does not offer blame nor praise, unasked-for sympathy in empty words and endless advice, will in most cases provide relief. Most especially should nurses be cautious when dealing with the difficulties that arise between husband and wife, for these are particularly common in psycho-neuroses, and she may very easibly be drawn into taking sides according to whether her natural or acquired sympathies incline her to the man's side or to that of the woman, so causing the breach between the two to be made wider at a time when emotional conflict is at its height.

It may not be amiss here to mention that some contraceptive methods may frequently undermine the nervous health of the man or the woman, as well as making emotional disturbances between them. But the details of these complications are the concern of the nerve specialist or the medical work of reference, rather than that of a more general nursing textbook, such as this aims to be.

One other important cause of both these kinds of neurosis in which guilt plays an important part, however, before passing on to the symptoms that take the form of physical illness. This is *masturbation*, commonly referred to as self-abuse or bad habits. In the past, and also now occasionally, we have heard or read warnings given that this will originate the most horrible diseases, or insanity, blindness, as well as neurasthenia. Modern research, however, has declared these threats to be without real physical basis, although instances are only too common when a condition resembling what has been threatened appears of psychological origin, created out of fear and guilt, due to the destructive suggestion and usually representing at the same time an attempt at self-punishment and atonement. The guilt arising from trying unsuccessfully to check the habit, and the conflict produced by the inability to prevent the wish to do so recurring, will often have been responsible for many neurotic conditions, which may sometimes be dispelled by some sound information on the subject, and, especially in the case of young people, should a clearer knowledge be gained of the functions of the body and of the physical and mental changes or readjustments of puberty.

Very frequent masturbation certainly drains physical energy in most cases, but then this is not a normal state of affairs, nor is the mental condition which brings it about, and the consequent exhaustion after arises from the mental conflict and guilt which becomes connected with it. Constant masturbation is in itself a sign that the child, adolescent or adult, is not getting something else that is necessary to their psychological well-being. The condition needs thorough investigation and treatment by an expert for the permanent relief of the patient, who may be reassured that this symptom can be alleviated and that the trouble is neither a sign of incipient insanity nor a token of moral imbecility.

One of the most important functions of the nurse with regard to psychological disorders is to re-educate the public respecting them, and by her own attitude and knowledge concerning their origin and scope to lead others to change their opinions, on the one hand, from believing them to be mere shams and an empty bid for sympathy or indulgence, on the other incurable madness or moral lapses beyond cure or sympathy.

An imagination that is diseased so that it cannot function properly is by no means less interesting than an organ of the body that is suffering from too great or too little ability to perform its special task, to the detriment of the whole body, and thus hindering the life capacity of its owner. It is more difficult to cure the mental process, certainly it is more elusive; but its diseases and their possibilities of treatment are now becoming more familiar to those who have made a special study of them, so that they are no longer the mysterious and baffling condition that they were in the past.

We have already remarked that several forms of *physical ill-health* will often be discernible in the neurasthenic, especially those that are connected with the gastro-intestinal tract. The patient appears to be suffering from acute malnutrition, accompanied often with constipation and flatulent dispepsia, and complains of feelings of revulsion when confronted by certain kinds of food. These cases are perhaps especially interesting to the nurse, and may call forth the exercise of much professional strategy before the situation may be effectually dealt with.

It may make these cases clearer should we begin by dividing the neurasthenia that arises from malnutrition into two main groups.

A. The patients whose nervous debility has been produced and the general vitality lowered through an actual insufficiency of food, or of sufficiently nourishing food, which has been caused by famine, illness, or to the economic difficulties of the person.

B. Those who have been reduced to the same condition, not because there has been any real necessity to deny the body the essentials of health, but because the patient wishes to do so for purposes of self-sacrifice or in consequence of some other morbid idea.

A. Patients of the first type are, nevertheless, only too numerous. In all our large cities, unfortunately, there are large numbers of middle-aged or elderly women eking out a miserable existence, and trying to keep up appearances upon a pittance that scarcely keeps them from starvation line, and certainly undermining their nervous health long before such an acute stage of deprivation is reached as to require hospital treatment. The fact that such deprivation is present and causes the gastro-intestinal symptoms is often overlooked. The patient complains of indigestion, which is actually the result of hunger, unhappiness, and the absence of all that makes life worth living. These cases may finally drift into hospital or the infirmary, and benefit by their stay there, but will soon relapse upon return to their wretched life of loneliness, somewhere high up in a tiny room, without interest or companionship.

The loveless lives lived by these people has contributed extensively to the distressing state of their neurosis. Starved emotions, together with a starved body, provide a forcing-ground for the graver mental disturbances which might never have gained an upper hand under more fortunate surroundings. They are apt to become suspicious, and melancholy also, frequently imagining that others are plotting against them, or that a large organisation is working for their ultimate relief. The prescription to deal adequately with the trouble would be a transformation by a magic wand to change their unhappy, lonely, and sordid existence into one of more normal home relationships; but it is a difficult change to bring about, because such persons will often regard any attempt to take a friendly interest in their troubles from the outside as unwarrantable interference, and treat the offer of any help in their loneliness as a direct insult.

The extreme reticence of these patients and their acute sensitiveness over their unhappy state, which they work so hard to keep secret, often makes them doubly hard to nurse. Moreover, the miserable life which lies ahead, when their stay in the hospital or other institution comes to an end, with its opportunity for human contacts, interest, and sympathy, makes recovery relatively slow, because of the operation of that mechanism that we have already described —the secondary gain of the illness. It is probable that the nurse may divine the real cause of the trouble in some instances before the doctor, and the warm-hearted woman cannot but regret that there is so little that can be done to relieve the real and most pressing cause of the symptoms, since help in any form and often even sympathy will be taken amiss, being thought of as the equivalent of charity and resented as such.

B. The second cause of malnutrition in neurasthenia is more difficult to understand, and also offers a less direct appeal to our natural sympathies. This is self-inflicted malnutrition in the midst of plenty, or when a sufficiency of food might be procured, which arises from a conscious or an unconscious reason. Cases of this sort frequently find their way into the columns of our newspapers, where some man or woman, living a solitary life, has been found at the point of death, or dead from deprivation, with a large sum of money hidden upon their person or with their mattress stuffed full of bank notes, so that poverty cannot have been the reason for this condition, but deliberate self-abnegation. Sometimes, however, without reaching such lengths as these, we will find that a patient will refuse all food prepared or brought by a certain person, or some kinds of food, which in special cases will be caused by a delusion or suspicion that poison is being administered or that the food is dirty. In other cases the refusal of nourishment will be maintained to alarm some near relative, who becomes anxious about the loss of appetite; as a demonstration of illness, or to prove unhappiness supposed to have been caused by another in the hope that this symptom may win sympathy and bring about contrition from this person, as well as occasionally from motives of revenge. These conditions may often play an important part in the psychological illness of young people, and revive the classical connection between loss of appetite and some disappointment in love.

We may also find, belonging to this type of patient, a wide array of food idiosyncrasies. Only a few food-stuffs of very doubtful nutritional value will be liked, and eaten, while others of real nutritional worth are said to cause nausea or vomiting. In some cases the patient will apparently eat scarcely anything at meal-times and to the knowledge of those who are looking after her, and secretly consume quite large quantities of somewhat unwholesome food. The nurse, whose lot it is to attempt to carry out the care of a patient of this type, will have her skill, knowledge, and ingenuity tried to the utmost. In the last type of apparent lost appetite we will naturally recall the case of the "secret drinker," and would be prepared to find a collection of interesting psychological reasons which account for each, were we able to trace both conditions to their source.

We are all familiar with feeding difficulties of all kinds connected with neuroses in the wards of our hospitals and similar institutions, where the food provided for the patients is a source of constant friction, sometimes even of hostility, on the part of the neurasthenic patients, who do not want to eat anything that has been prepared in the hospital. They wish to have everything sent in from home, or the bone of contention may be that food that others are eating seems particularly unpalatable. It will be said to be badly cooked, or that the spoons or forks have not been properly washed and are dirty, so that something may be "caught from another patient" who is not *clean*. Specially are they unwilling to eat what is provided for all the inmates of the ward in common, and will do their utmost to be placed upon some special diet. Should the attempt be successful they will become quite cheerful, although getting better becomes a complex problem, since recovery includes being able to return to ordinary diet. So the recuperation is obliged to remain carefully just below the level of return to share the food of the others. It will be particularly pleasing to these patients should one of the nurses or the Sister of the ward herself become responsible for the administration of the special diet or its preparation for this reason: this dislike of sharing common food often belongs to a complex, which, for want of a better name, may be called *snobbishness*. We will frequently find that feelings of this sort become more plainly indicated over food than in many other ways. Fastidiousness will in this case be regarded as a sign of gentle birth and breeding, and being unable to eat what the other patients are expected to consume provides a hint to the nursing staff that this patient is not accustomed to such plebeian fare. All these many little complexities of the attempt to set up a social pedestal will be so familiar to the nurse that it is hardly necessary to explain the outward signs of the type further. Frequently, however, this desire for something different covers another of a rather more remote and not so obvious nature, which probably accounts for the superficial manifestations that we have been describing—namely, the struggle to establish marks of distinction between the self and the rest of the community, which is such a general element in the neurosis. (See Chapters V and VI.)

It is quite interesting to watch the influence of the minds of these patients upon the process of digestion and metabolism, since the results of their hostility to some idea thus becomes visible in their state of physical malnutrition. The food disagrees with them in the same manner as they are in disharmony with somebody or the world at large, which conflict allows them to accept nothing. We may often find the origin of this condition in infancy, which is repeated during life. We will offer a more detailed explanation of the causes of these awkward conditions in the chapter dealing with the neuroses of children, and pass on now to suggest a few guiding hints for the nursing of these perplexing patients.

One of the most important points to keep in view is this, that the failure to ingest or digest food so that it provides nourishment for the body may frequently represent a failure to obtain *love* in some form or another. We are out of love with some other person, with ourselves, or with life in general. Should we deliberate upon the earliest experiences of taking nourishment, which is one of the most important preoccupations and pleasures of infant life, we will find that food, mother, and love are so intimately connected that to the baby's rudimentary mind at that stage they are practically identical.

The child gradually becomes aware of the love of the mother during the reception of food. The reverse, a withholding of food by the mother, or its own refusal of food, will produce feelings in the child to which it will afterwards attach such meanings as unhappiness or hatred. Both these ideas will be intimately connected with that of hunger, so that the reverse situation will also occur, the refusal of food, should anything have upset the love of the child for the usual provider of nourishment, or should some other circumstances have caused unhappiness. The absence of a loved person who has been associated in the child's mind with the administration of food is often a signal for a period of malnutrition or refusal of food throughout life, or the failure of proper assimilation of the nutriment even if swallowed as usual, which is none the less a refusal and produces the same result—emaciation. The baby who goes on hunger-strike and thus forces authorities to capitulate by the restoration of the accustomed person or food, as sometimes happens in connection with weaning difficulties, will always show this same tendency in later life to attempt a similar strategy to enforce compliance with his or her wishes.

Keeping this in mind, the nurse may proceed cautiously with the feeding of her neurasthenic patients. She may score a point as a provider of food because she comes fresh into her patient's environment and will therefore be free from the immediate former hostility that has been attached to others in the administration of food, but may still encounter this difficulty if an old association linger on in the mind of this patient concerning a tendency to refuse food from a stranger, which we find in some infants. The attitude of the nurse and the suggestion implied by it nevertheless plays a significant part, for it is one that expects compliance with her wishes; and if in addition to this her patient should take a fancy to her from the start, things will probably go smoothly until some fresh set of troubles appear from depths in the patient's unconscious mind.

The fact that a patient will often take food from the nurse when it has formerly been refused from members of the household will often produce comments of some asperity, such as these, which lead us to suppose that these matters are the cause of no little jealousy in the household where the arrival of the nurse to take over the reins of government are concerned: "I cannot think why you can so easily get the patient to take the nourishment that has been ordered. We have tried in all ways, and have found it quite useless." The patient's quarrel in this case had probably been with the people who brought or prepared the food, now it is in the hands of another person the whole situation has been drained of hostility.

The nurse who can gain a rapid transference from her

patient, to whom, in common parlance, the patient takes a fancy at first sight, has already gone far towards winning the battle with the neurotic case, provided she knows what to do with it when she has it, which is by no means always the case. The transference, caused by her charm of manner, her appearance, and her attitude of sympathy, will arise partly from natural endowment and partly from her knowledge both of herself and the structure of the illness before her. This enables the sick person gradually to wish to exchange the former condition of illness, which was providing some sort of gratification, although generally unrecognised by the patient, for health, in imitation of the nurse, as well as to give her the pleasure of effecting the cure. We often find in cases of persistent illness that the patient unconsciously does not want to get well, because he or she grudges to give this credit to doctor or nurse. This being the case, another important nursing principle is put into our hands: that the breaking down of the transference between nurse and patient, or the change from the positive (the attitude of liking, such as we have described) to the negative (where the patient's dislike or hate is aroused instead of love), unless skilfully handled, will lead to protracted illness or the exchange of the nurse.

Much of the trouble will actually arise from the unconscious attitude of the nurse towards her patients and their relations. The nurse, who consciously or unconsciously does not like "nerve cases," or who considers them tiresome, uncontrolled, and that they give her unnecessary trouble, will with certainty stimulate the hostility of her patients, so making impossible for them to allow themselves to be brought to health by her, because this would mean giving her too much sway over them, or add more than they wish to her professional reputation. Their hatred of her, or of the mother-figure, whom the nurse nearly always represents, even if the idea remains unconscious, would tend to make them resist her, unless in rare cases the only way to rid themselves of her unwanted presence and ministrations seemed to be to recover their health so that they could once more do without her.

One more difficulty in achieving the recovery of the patient suffering from a nervous disorder arises from the unconscious wishes of the nurse who has gained a positive transference from her patient. The patient loves the nurse so much that parting with her becomes unbearable. In this case the nurse may be deriving an equal satisfaction from looking after this helpless invalid. The trouble therefore remains chronic, and the nurse a permanent institution because she is now both physically and psychologically indispensable to her patient's well-being. Recovery may also be hindered if the nurse prefers her helpless patients. Unconscious mind may communicate with another unconscious mind without any verbal explanation taking place, and the child that remains in the patient readily responds to the mother wish in the nurse to tend the helpless.

The unconscious mechanism by which the patient places the nurse in the rôle of the mother is one of the greatest importance for all nursing, but particularly so in the case of those suffering from psycho-neuroses. In these patients we nearly always find that the original attitude towards this parent played an overwhelming part for later life, whether it was through a love-fixation to her influence, because of which the child has never been able subsequently to reach complete adult independence, or through hatred of her, which has warped all other social relationships throughout life. The conditions of illness, when once the sick person returns to a childish state of dependence upon a woman, be it mother or nurse, will revive all the old associations of childhood, as well as the childish behaviour that was once connected with this period of life. Should we carefully watch the reactions of the invalid, the connections between them and childhood are not difficult to observe; and we may generally rely upon hearing sooner or later some recollections of early illnesses or spans of ill-health, when the mother or nursery-nurse had to neglect other duties or persons in order to concentrate exclusively upon this one little patient.

When such has been the case in the past we will usually find a particularly childish dependence upon the ministrations of the nurse, a helpless clinging to her support, with frequent appeals for sympathy, which will be required in some definite form of demonstrative affection or assurances of her preference, and continued assistance as long as it should be required.

Since the patient has psychologically returned to childhood for the period of the illness, we cannot expect otherwise than that the behaviour will keep pace with the degree of the regression. The mind and its working will also follow along the same line, so that adult reasoning and logic fall completely into abeyance. This naturally accounts for the caprice and unreliability that we all recognise as typical of sick folk, and is especially prevalent in nervous troubles. It is for this reason that the gastro-intestinal tract plays its prominent part in neurasthenia, for it is the essential physical process of early childhood and of infancy which consequently leaves an indelible trace upon the mind of the child in due proportion.

The infant's earliest interests and preoccupations lie in this direction; its fluctuations of bodily health, emotional well-being, and life in general centre around this tract between the mouth and the anus, the intake of food and the expulsion of its residue. Those of us who have studied the ways of infants to any extent will readily endorse this view, and will recognise that the neurasthenic returns to the same interests as a preoccupation taking precedence of all others—namely, food and the action of the intestines.

These two subjects frequently absorb the entire mental outlook of such patients, and they contemplate nothing all the day long but the comparative nutritional values of foods, their digestibility, and the topic of constipation, which represents the second stage of paramount interest and pleasure to the infant—the evacuation of its bowels. The subject of constipation might even be regarded as the most popular hobby of the present day, should we consider the amount of literature and publicity that are given to it, showing how readily adults will seize any opportunity of returning to one of the main interests of their childhood, which later became taboo, and therefore repressed, yet at the same time remained waiting for any chance to find expression that would be compatible with social standards.

The infant's food and bowel habits both show the same tendency to become permanent, and all exhibit a similar aspect in their intimate connection with other persons who first confronted the infant with ideas of training and discipline in relation to these two functions. This external control of its wishes aroused in the infant feelings representing more or less hostility and forced upon its recognition the possibility of an environment that did not necessarily comply with all its desires. Before birth we may assume that such a state of affairs was impossible, and that the baby's mind contained no wish, since this implies a recognised need. At that stage of development everything requisite for the baby's comfort was automatically supplied, and its activities were unrestrained, except perhaps spatially, which was probably never realised at the time as a limitation caused by the presence of another. It is only post-natally that the infant is faced with the proposition of an opposing will, against which it may struggle, or with the demands of which it must comply.

The history of this struggle or compliance is one that is extremely interesting and far-reaching, setting its seal upon the subsequent life of the individual. It may be observed with the greatest prominence in these conditions of psycho-genic illness, because the personality for some reason became fixated at one of these early stages of development with the concomitant food, bowel, or bladder disturbances connected with the original attitude of the baby towards the people who first ministered to its comfort or to discipline in these respects.

We have already discussed some of the problems and difficulties that arise in relation to feeding the neurotic patient, and our thoughts reviewing the behaviour or interest of other patients concerning bowel action will probably corroborate the second half of the proposition, that in this respect also the patient is equally the child, showing as much interest, compliance, defiance, or obstinacy as the infant itself or the young child.

The patient, who in infancy was compliant and easily adapted itself to the ideas of those responsible for its training in these matters, gives little or no trouble in this way when ill, but we find a different state of affairs should we encounter one who struggled to maintain his or her own prerogative in the matter of bowel function. These are the patients who are troubled with chronic constipation more or less severe, and we usually remark corresponding and characteristic obstinacy, defiance, and unwillingness to relinquish anything else that belongs to them at the instigation of another, in these same persons.

The child who, when very young, met strong counter-opposition in this respect, will show greater resistance than the one trained by gentler methods, and it is by no means infrequent to find adults aroused to keen demonstrations of emotion and showing emotional reactions towards the infant who offers protracted resistance to their training in this respect. Both adult and infant exhibit an equal dislike of being beaten in this contest of wills, but the adult usually wins through power to administer strong purgatives, or that still more deadly weapon, so injurious to the child's later character-development, the enema or rectal injection. Children who have been early accustomed to these strong measures tend to act only when compelled by a *force majeure.* They will show a lack of personal initiative, and yet store up an immense reserve of hatred towards the person who has thus overcome them.

In some cases, however, especially in male children, this action may have aroused a certain amount of erotic feelings even in infancy, so that they will later on still continue to derive considerable gratification from ministrations of this kind from the nurse, doing their best, consciously or unconsciously, to render this treatment necessary, a contingency to which the eyes of the nurse should be open, so that she may circumvent the gratification of the enema whenever possible. Should this wish become too strong it could easily be a cause of constipation.

The interest of the child that originally was discovered by the adult responsible for its training to be too persistently centred upon bowel action was usually sternly repressed, more or less guilt being consequently attached to the matter as the means to the end of shifting the focus of attention. Because the child failed to show outwardly a continuance of the interest, it does not follow that this ceased to exist, which is often fondly believed by the educating authority. The matter is kept to itself for the future, it continues the preoccupation in secret, accepts the guilt that becomes attached to it, and stores up its dislike against the people who have thwarted its pleasure and interest. Hate soon takes as its companion Fear of the adults in the environment, and these three psychological factors, Guilt, Hatred, and Fear, continue to weave an intricate pattern of nervous symptoms in the life of the person in whom they have gained a firm hold, so that at any time they may appear upon the surface in definite illness.

If the earlier stages of infancy contribute these origins of nervous trouble that concern the *oral side* of the gastro-intestinal symptoms and may be seen in the food idiosyncrasies, malnutrition and gastric inhibitions, otherwise the flatulent dispepsia of the neurasthenic that involve the upper regions of the alimentary canal, the lower section of this tract is responsible for a wide range of intestinal ailments and abnormalities to which many names and origins are ascribed. For these also the recrudescence of old conditions of infant hostility is responsible, and we will frequently find them allocated among the symptoms of neurasthenia. They are, however, naturally very closely associated with those characteristic of hypochondria.

Actually, nevertheless, we may often remark with the transition of focus of attention down the gastro-intestinal tract a change from the symptoms usually connected with neurasthenia to those of the obsessional neurosis, except to the extent of the syndromes which arise from extreme bowel inactivity. Constipation may thus arise from two main causes: *extreme feebleness or lassitude of peristalsis*, comparable with the general nervous exhaustion of the neurasthenic, or from *muscular opposition to peristalsis*, typical of the hostility and hatred caused by the struggle against all natural promptings, as against those of the mother, which would all lead to the same result of constipation, through the unconscious resistance of peristalsis, or, indeed, muscular action that we usually regard as involuntary may possibly be controlled by the unconscious mind. Certainly the resistance and opposition of the patient controls the anal sphincters with the same result—withholding the stool. These muscles respond vigorously to the wish of opposition in the youngest infant, as anyone soon discovers in the nursing of these small patients.

Obsessional Neuroses

Let us now turn to a brief study of the obsessional neuroses, although usually these patients do not so often come into the care of the nurse with general training as do those suffering from neurasthenia, because in the more advanced stages the symptoms are so closely related to the psychotic conditions that the patients may require the shelter of a mental hospital, or a nurse with mental training will be called into look after them, should they stay at home. Yet it is not uncommon to find those with slight manifestations of this disease among our patients or even in the ranks of those who consider themselves quite normal, and only pass as "rather odd!" among their friends and relations.

Dr. Ernest Jones, in his chapter on this subject in *Treatment of the Neuroses* (Baillière, Tindall & Cox), gives as the diagnosis condition the "feeling of mustness" which compels the patient to carry out certain actions, generally in a particular way. Sometimes the exact number of times that the actions must be performed is of importance, at others the special method to be observed is of greater significance. But whatever variations we may find in the procedure, the compulsive nature of the action or thought remains, also the acute mental distress which arises should any interruption occur to prevent the ritual being completed, or should someone try to restrain the habit. The distress is typical of the condition, although connected with actions that seem trivial, or even ridiculous in some cases to those who do not understand their significance. Frequently these patients themselves do not realise the true meaning of their obsessions, nor of their origin, but when we have become conversant with these we remark that the emotion which their performance arouses is quite comparable with the danger they are often supposed to avert. Usually they concern severe injury or even the death of someone dear to the patient, and are accompanied by feelings of intense guilt and fear, which points to the fact that the third companion of this trio, hatred of this same person who is so tenderly loved, is not far distant in the unconscious, and provides this defence mechanism, so that the unconsciously wished harm may be atoned for simultaneously.

Another feature usually to be observed in these compulsive actions is that some detail of the routine represents or repeats a fragment of an emotionally toned scene of the past that has remained stamped in the mind. The scene is thus reiterated in the hope somehow of obliterating or atoning for this guilty memory, although usually this remnant is all that survives, the rest having been dragged down into the unconscious through the action of repression. We are reminded in connection with the obsessional neurosis of the constantly repeated action of Lady Macbeth, in which she appears washing her hands during her sleep-walking, trying symbolically to cleanse the stain from her conscience.

It is interesting to note that this obsession is one that may frequently be met, especially in women, in varying degrees, from scrupulosity about the cleansing of hands and household utensils to the fully developed mania, which gives the patient little rest from torturing doubt whether the rituals of ablution have been correctly performed, so that they must be repeated again and again until the hands are sore and disfigured with infinite applications of the strongest disinfectant soap and very hot water.

The element of Doubt always plays a significant part in these obsessional neuroses, and the patient will seek from the nurse, or any other person regarded as an authority, repeated reassurance that all is well, that the ritual has been satisfactorily carried out and need not be repeated. The over-conscientious housewife shows some of these same symptoms as the obsessional neurotic, a certain routine must be carried out correctly in every detail, or she is miserable and feels guilty of having committed an unpardonable sin of neglect. These obsessions and rituals may be applied to practically any action of daily life, and there are few persons who do not show some trace of the same tendency. Some of the most common are the rituals associated with getting up, going to bed, bathing, and in other persons of attending to the excretory functions.

It is impossible to remain oblivious of this close connection between the exaggerated rôle played by cleanliness, method, and conscientiousness in the obsessional neurosis, together with its fear of contamination by dirt and disease, with the emphasis placed upon *doing* and *not doing*, and the excretory function. In childhood this subject becomes inevitably associated with the idea *dirty* or *rude*, and the words *doing something*, or even *business*, have likewise a double meaning of the same description. When we come to discover the origins of these serious nervous conditions we usually find primal conflicts of this kind, and that adults in charge of the training of the baby placed too much emphasis on *perfect cleanliness* being acquired too soon, or inculcated them with over-severe measures, teaching the child extreme guiltiness about any lapse in this direction, which survives and finds a revival of affect in the obsessional symptoms.

The sick person often shows us some of these tendencies during the process of another disease, when toilet or other matters are carried out with meticulous precision and sleep is impossible unless certain articles are first deposited in an habitual resting-place. Thus candle and matches maybe must be laid on a corner of a table, pulled up beside the bed. In one case a man could not sleep until his watch was placed in a box, wrapped up in cotton-wool, so that he could not hear it ticking, which kept him awake. A box of biscuits must always be near at hand in case of sudden hunger, chairs must be pulled out from the wall and pillows placed in some peculiar fashion, then and then only may sleep be induced. Other patients carry out elaborate preparations before letters can be opened and read or written, money handled, or meals partaken of.

We are reminded thus in many ways of the customs that are associated with the rituals of religion and magic, once in the world's history so closely connected. Many years ago now Freud called attention to this relation between ancient magic rituals and the symptoms of neurotic patients, and remarked that they were particularly common among persons suffering from obsessional neurosis, who are always trying thus to atone for or avoid some real or imaginary wrong-doing, and who, instead of actually feeling guilty, merely feel ill. (See *Totem and Taboo*. Sigmund Freud. Trans. George Allen & Unwin.)

The "mustness" which is connected with obsessional neurosis may refer to various groups of human activities, which may be tabulated as follows:

A. *Motor Group*, in which the obsession refers to actions that must either be carried out in some special way by the patient almost as rituals, a lapse of even the smallest detail in which would involve the patient or others in serious danger, or which must be entirely refrained from for the same reason—a consequent penalty.

B. *Sensory Group*, effects sensations or obsessive hallucinations connected with any of the special senses.

C. *Ideational*. Comprises mental obsessions or thoughts often of an infantile character, sometimes also blasphemous or obscene, which are connected in the mind of the patient with feelings of extreme horror and guilt. This group is often closely allied with B, because the thoughts may be projected externally by the patient, who will then hear them as voices, in which they become equivalent to an auditory hallucination.

D. *Affective*. These are the obsessive emotions, love, hatred, fear, which are felt to be compulsory under certain conditions known only to the patient. Although he or she may realise that these are quite unreasonable, or without due foundation, they still continue to exert their power over many of the functions of life, both on the side of action as well as in the limitation of action, which produces the inhibition.

The symptoms which belong to this last group will be hard to distinguish from those that are usually placed among the forms of anxiety hysteria, for many reasons, unless we hold rigidly to the criterion of their compulsive character, through which the fear will be responsible for some action or inhibition as a defence mechanism. The form of obsessive fear that mainly concerns the nurse will be when the focus has been placed upon some disease, and takes the form that the patient is obsessed with the idea that he or she is (i) suffering with it at the time, (ii) will contract it in the future, (iii) or that someone else has it and so must consequently be avoided.

The nurse will usually be able to recall to mind some patients who have come under her observation with symptoms of this kind, even should they not have been the actual cause of her presence. Yet, although a mild degree of obsession is frequently looked upon as merely an idiosyncrasy, their more severe forms often give rise to the opinion that the patient is suffering from mental rather than neurotic trouble, and consequently becomes the charge of nurses with medico-psychological training rather than those who have gained their certificates in general hospitals. It is complications of this kind which cause thinking persons in the nursing world to feel that the day has come when the two types of training should not be kept so rigidly apart, and that both schools should in some way transfer the knowledge imparted to their students to those trained or in training in the sister institutions. The line of demarcation is frequently so very tenuous between physical and mental sickness that in the near future it is quite possible that we may see the three great branches of Medicine, Surgery, and Psychology, working closely together in co-operation, without splitting up the training into such water-tight compartments.

With the increase in severity of these symptoms the ordinary conditions of life become extremely difficult, and for these patients to continue to reside with their families or with others who have no special knowledge or understanding of their condition is almost impossible. What to do with them is a complicated problem, nevertheless. Unless treated at an early stage by some person and method adequate to relieve their distress, it is extremely doubtful that their condition will recover spontaneously. If, however, the patient's family can bear the strain financially, the situation is often met by installing a permanent nurse and arranging special quarters in the house, equipped to provide for carrying out, without interruption, the special rituals and conditions of the neurosis. But we must realise that this procedure can hardly be expected *to cure* the abnormal state of the patient. All that may be hoped from it is to prevent avoidable distress for the patient, and conflict with normal people, who would be worried by the symptoms, through the segregation and the provision of this unreal environment made to accommodate these symptomatic rituals, unless a course of treatment were undertaken at the same time, when in due course the special conditions of life might once more be relinquished and replaced by the ordinary routine of daily life.

Otherwise, what can become of such patients without provision of an adequate cure? Medicine cannot mend matters in this case, and surgery is helpless to alter their condition. The ordinary nursing-home, for this same reason, does not want them. The general hospital certainly cannot fill its beds with these chronic cases, nor do the specialised hospitals or homes care for patients of this type, since they are typically inclined to involve others in their obsessions, which makes nursing them with other patients extremely difficult. Often they drift eventually into our asylums or mental hospitals, where only too frequently nothing definite is done by way of treatment or cure, and their problems are solved for the time being merely through the expedient of preventing them unduly worrying the general public with their uncomfortable or peculiar symptoms. But naturally this does not provide a real solution to the problem of the obsessional neurotic, that can only be accomplished when we provide a means of cure.

The nurse alone can do little towards a radical cure for this condition, which might be compared to a major operation, only to be attempted by a skilled and experienced operator, since it is one of great severity. Still, she can help to relieve the patient's distress meanwhile by her understanding of the possible difficulties that are causing the conflict in the mind of this person suffering from obsessions. This knowledge will also be of assistance to her in dealing with situations that arise and call for more than ordinary tact, that are well calculated to cause perplexity for all who have no specialised information about what may be represented by the strange requirements and actions of these patients, which neither ordinary nursing knowledge nor skill can provide.

These people will often demand the co-operation of the nurse in carrying out their obsessional rituals, and the problem will emerge, to what extent is it best to comply with these requests, or to refuse, in cases where the action in itself is one of no great moment to the nurse. Whenever possible she should try to get into communication with the doctor carrying out the treatment of the patient and ascertain as far as may be the importance or significance of this co-operation for the patient, and what his instructions are in this respect. In some forms of obsessional neurosis the patient will need assistance occasionally to help carry on in some especially difficult crises, and the refusal of help might impose a strain upon the mental condition that would actually be unwise or dangerous. At other times the necessity of facing the difficulty might cause material to be remembered or brought to light in the treatment which otherwise would never appear, should the patient be receiving too much comfort and palliation for the symptom through the help and sympathy of the nurse, since this would supply direct gratification and act as a defence against the fear represented and guarded against by the action.

The nurse is as necessary to the doctor during the treatment of these severe neurotic cases as in the after-treatment of major abdominal operations or pneumonia, and it is only through close co-operation that both may gain an adequate understanding of the case. The nurse, who is in constant attendance upon the daily life of the patient, may be able to contribute much information from her observation that the doctor might not otherwise hear from the patient; while the nurse will be greatly helped by some account from the medical man of the unconscious processes at work that are causing the symptoms which she observes and with which she has to deal throughout the day and night.

Thus it is by no means uncommon for the obsessional patient, instead of continually wanting to clean out and throw away all rubbish and the contents of cupboards and drawers, to refuse to have them touched, or perhaps to have the bed made, for fear of spreading contamination. Yet others will require certain articles of clothing or draperies about the room or house destroyed in special ways, should they feel them to have become polluted. It is easy to see that if all these ideas were carried out by the nurse an awkward situation might arise. On the other hand, in some cases the refusal of the nurse to comply with *any* request would cause the sick person unnecessary distress and provoke anxiety attacks which may have serious consequences, although in all probability they would not, since the threat of an anxiety attack is a defence by which many neurotic patients manage to rule his or her environment.

It is in cases such as these that the nurse requires particular and explicit instructions for the case in question from the doctor in charge, and then it is up to her to carry them out, as in nursing any other acute disease. She should, however, be on her guard against the following contingency. The obsessional patient, in accordance with the origins of this form of disease, will often try to play off father against mother, repeating some old situation from childhood: mother now represented by the nurse and father by the doctor. Concessions will be obtained if possible, one will be cajoled, threatened, or treated with indifference to obtain what is wanted, or to arouse the jealousy or sympathy of the other. Neither doctor nor nurse should permit themselves to be tricked into playing the part that is required by the patient; but it must be remembered that the methods are frequently so subtle and the unconscious of the patient so cleverly adjusts them to the most susceptible spot of the other's psychological make-up that it is not infrequent that the patient wins, and the doctor and the nurse fall into line without realising until too late that they have done so.

Never for one instant should the nurse in charge of the obsessional patient forget the fact that this nervous trouble seldom afflicts the foolish or unintelligent man, woman, or child, although some of the obsessions themselves may on the surface appear to the initiated as so childish. Nursing all kinds of nervous disease calls for the greatest intelligence on the side of the nurse, the keenest observation and foresight, but in no other so much general acumen as in this. The woman, especially, who suffers from obsessional neurosis is usually far from being a mental degenerate, and will easily outwit the nurse of no particular mental ability; and for this reason these cases offer the more interest to the intellect of the nurse, who is keen enough to grapple with the situation and make herself acquainted with the underlying principles of it.

Once or twice already we have mentioned the term

Anxiety or *Anxiety State*, without any special description of what is meant by it. The condition varies in degree of intensity from anxious or fearful expectation, often accompanied by trembling, sweating, the wish to urinate, or a feeling of dryness in the mouth, through all stages until one that approaches a frenzy of fear is reached, when all these signs occur greatly magnified, with the addition of the sensation of suffocation, or air hunger, and often of imminent death. Once we have had occasion to witness an anxiety attack we shall instantly recognise it again, unless the degree is unusually slight and under the control of the patient. We shall then remark that the anxiety portrayed is real enough for the patient, although to the onlooker the external provocative cause may seem entirely inadequate. The most severe attacks of this kind will often be found connected with a fear of death and may appear in patients during the night preceding an operation or during pregnancy, but are also by no means uncommon in men and women who are in normal physical health or only slightly indisposed physically, and where the danger of a fatal termination to their illness is quite unlikely.

Anxiety may cause many undesirable complications of other physical complaints, chief among which, perhaps, is insomnia, which will increase the nurse's difficulties to a very great extent. It will make night nursing in such cases particularly onerous, since all forms of narcotic drugs or sedatives may be entirely without effect, or merely produce broken sleep often made unbearable because of the presence of terrifying anxiety dreams, through which state of affairs sleep will become dreaded by the patient, and from which he or she will wake in a panic, bathed in sweat and fearing to sleep again lest they should reappear. One will see that this being the case, restful nights are out of the question, although rest is one of the great essentials of recovery. However, by means of these same alarming dreams we may often gain valuable clues to the real cause of the anxiety, and should the patient supply us with any account of them it is worth while to keep a record of them to be given to the doctor at the earliest opportunity, together with any special observations upon occurrences of the previous day that seemed to make a special impression upon the patient or any remarkable position assumed by the patient in sleep, or of any incontinence of any sort. This is always a possibility during an anxiety dream or attack, and should always be noted and reported. It is perhaps unnecessary to mention that reports of this description for the medical man should always be transferred to him without the knowledge of the patient, nor should it be known that the nurse is making any special observations of the case other than those connected with the usual nursing routine of keeping clinical charts to which the patient is accustomed.

The dream state of patients suffering from neurotic illness is always important, since it is closely allied to the undercurrent of their mental processes, which reach the surface in the obsessional actions, hallucinations, thoughts, and fears into which we have grouped the symptoms of this form of neurosis. Freud has called the dream the "highroad to the Unconscious," and if we take the trouble to study them, we shall find they give us some interesting information that we should not have obtained otherwise in most instances.

One other factor which often takes a prominent part in obsessional neurosis is what will be called *dissociation of personality* in textbooks upon nervous disease, because the patient not infrequently imagines that these strange conditions are prompted, if not entirely caused, by some outside agency, some voice or a vague influence, occasionally in more advanced cases ascribed to an evil spirit or the devil. This form of neurosis we may identify with the conditions described as that of demoniacal possession, when the person would suddenly be compelled to acts of violence or strange, wild behaviour, quite at variance with his usual character, for which the onlookers as well as the sufferer were quite at a loss to account.

One will often hear these patients who are grievously tormented with obsessional thoughts uttering them aloud in a strained voice, quite different from their own, or perhaps arguing in two distinct voices against these hints, insinuations, and threats that are thus put forward. The patient will be convinced that these hallucinations are real at the time, but usually has intervals when it can be recognised that they are unlikely. When this realisation is altogether lost the condition of the patient's mind more nearly approaches psychosis, and may be termed insanity, although in reality the dividing line between severe obsessional neurosis and mania is a thin one, and the patient often has periods of relief when the symptoms seem to have disappeared altogether, followed by an increase of the obsessions when residence in a mental home is advisable for many reasons. In women this exacerbation of the symptoms will usually coincide with the cumulative tension that precedes the menstrual flow, which the nurse should note carefully, so as to be prepared for the next recurrence in advance. But this question will be discussed in greater detail when we reach the chapter on the nursing of women's nervous troubles.

CHAPTER IV

THE NEUROSES OF CHILDHOOD

The preceding chapters have already shown the origin of neurosis in childhood, and suggested that some abnormal conditions may have been visible in the child at an early age; but it is now our concern to inquire to what extent we may find actual neurotic manifestations in young children, whether they show similar symptoms or those recognisable as typical of adult neuroses, or if they should merely be summed up under the general term *nervousness* at that age.

At the present day it is by no means uncommon to hear mothers or nurses who talk of "nervy" babies, who show signs of restlessness, irritability, and fear even in infancy. They become easily upset in their sleeping habits, the taking of food, and the action of their bowels with very little physical cause, and often as the result of some emotional derangement, i.e. anger or grief. This condition will be attributed by some to an emotional disturbance of the mother during the pregnancy or to bad management of the infant after birth. Which factor played the greater part in the child's disposition to nervous instability it is hard to determine, but the probability is that both contributed their own share to the results.

PRENATAL INFLUENCES AND THOSE OF BIRTH

Some psychologists suggest that prenatal influences affect the later life of the child to an important extent; but at present the scanty material upon this subject which is available scarcely puts us in a position to make any definite statements upon exact causes and effects yet, although the evidence which has been gained is certainly in its favour. The experience of Birth also offers debatable ground as the possible starting-place for neurosis, especially those that show a preponderance of anxiety. Otto Rank, a Viennese psycho-analyst now working in Paris, has devoted a book, *Das Trauma der Geburt* (The Birth-Trauma), to this problem. In this little volume he follows up an early theory of Freud, that it is this tremendous event in the life of the child which gives rise to the constellation of discomforts that are all regarded as the typical symptoms of anxiety in later life. In support of this theory we should recall the ancient belief that children who were born by Cæsarian section grew up without knowing fear, and it would be interesting to know whether contemporary experience of such children confirms the old superstition. (*Das Trauma der Geburt.* Dr. Otto Rank. Int. Psychoanalytischer Verlag. Wien.)

One is inclined to believe that one finds a larger proportion of these *nervy* babies among those who have been the first-born, especially in cases where the mother was young and inexperienced of life and what marriage involved, unprepared for the responsibilities of motherhood, and apprehensive during the pregnancy concerning the future of herself and the child to come. This theory may gain support from the fact that we find the most happy, placid babies as the offspring of mothers who were tranquil and well-pleased with the idea of bringing a tiny life into the world, and the most miserable, restless infants as the result of unwished-for pregnancies. Between the two extremes, where the two factors obviously agree with results, we may nevertheless find many conflicting variations of cause and effect, which make conclusions the more difficult, since we are unable with any degree of certainty to ascertain the real thoughts that existed at that time in the mother's unconscious mind concerning the advent of the infant before or after its birth. This would be of even more importance than to learn her conscious thoughts.

It is, however, an accepted fact that the persons who

are in charge of infants during the first months of life have a permanent influence upon their subsequent character and habits, as well as their health, as every nurse is aware, who tries to impress the importance of this early stage upon the mother before she leaves at the end of her month. But the influence she is thinking about is usually that which she knows she is exerting. Usually she does not take into consideration that which is conveyed through her personality, as well as her conscious and unconscious tendencies in dealing with others, about which she often knows only too little. She is always ready to accept as her own training of the infant all its early virtues, good habits, and health, as the result of her ministrations, but usually is not willing to accept any responsibility for adverse manifestations. These one might imagine, from information gathered from the nurse or the mother, should she be looking after the infant herself, to be the unfortunate consequence of someone else's actions, or an inheritance from the father's side of the family. Yet, if we are going to be quite just, we ought to attribute the babies "vices" to the same source as its "virtues."

We are at present beginning to discover that unconscious tendencies on the part of the nurse, or others in close contact with an infant, will leave their mark upon the subsequent character in addition to the nervous health of the child. Any inclination to neurosis in the adult will rapidly be communicated to infants in their environment, such as restlessness, fussiness, undue anxiety, or apprehensiveness. Those persons training an infant, who are possessed of exaggerated ideas of the importance of trifles, or disproportionate insistence upon the correct following of a timetable with the rigidity of methods typical of the obsessional neurotic, sow seeds of future psychogenic trouble of the same description in the child. These meticulous observances show particularly clearly in respect to feeding habits and the training in cleanliness, to which we shall refer later on in this chapter.

The first baby is certainly greatly handicapped, inasmuch as it is a novelty, which often means that it is treated as a plaything by the mother, or she will be desperately afraid of it. Both are equally injurious to the emotional stability of the infant, who needs a tranquil existence for several months at least after birth, so as the difference between that state and its prenatal condition should not be too strongly marked. Noise, too much handling and excitement, are all predisposing causes of nervous unrest in babies and young children.

The apprehensiveness of a young mother, who is afraid of insufficient intellectual response on the part of the infant during its first few months, often makes her persistently try to force it to take notice of herself and other objects around long before its length of vision has developed sufficiently to enable it to do so. Her inexperience of what may fairly be expected from the baby makes her worry that things are not going on rightly, or not fast enough, and so she tries to increase the pace; but her action is as bad for the baby as that of the anxious little girl who digs up her seeds or plants in the garden to see if they have started to grow. Both manifestations come from the same source—impatience, and fear as well as doubt concerning her own ability to be a perfect producer of babies or gardens.

For this reason, that only experience can give us real self-confidence, it is always good when these first babies can be looked after by someone from the start who has had enough experience to be quite sure of her own ability and the methods she employs to be able to counteract the uncertainty of the mother and her anxiety. Given a mother with her first baby and a nurse with her first case on her own coinciding, the outlook for the psychological equilibrium of the infant would be meagre. The same difficulty, of course, holds good concerning the lack of experience in the nurse; self-confidence can only be gained with time, practice, and success, and the nurse also, in the early stages of her career, not uncommonly worries and overdoes things for fear of leaving undone something that may be very important, but it is not conducive to the nervous health of her patients.

Feeding and Weaning

The next definite danger-point at which neurotic troubles of childhood may arise is that of Feeding and Weaning. We are fully aware of the obvious difficulties that may arise over this process, especially if the illness or enforced absence of the mother, as well as her aversion, make it necessary to resort to artificial foods or to weaning before the usual time. It will also be apparent that the infant's reactions to a premature weaning vary considerably, since one will submit to the substitution with very little hesitation, while others show clear and bitter resentment, resisting to the utmost, sometimes compelling the return of the favourite food for a time for fear of the consequences otherwise.

Those of us who have had the opportunity to investigate cases of child or adult neuroses constantly find that these early difficulties are reflected in the subsequent symptoms or obsessional ideas of their patients. Thus one will perpetually complain that *the whole world seems to conspire to do him out of his rights, that he cannot and will not put up with substitutes.* Or another will bemoan the fact that she *never realised how well off she was until she was deprived of something.* It is by no means uncommon to find people experiencing extreme disgust or horror when they see a human mother or even an animal suckling her baby, and may feel that they wish to destroy or injure the little one because it looks so blissfully content. In rare cases the feeling becomes so strong that a sudden exclamation may reveal the truth, and the root of the matter will be put into words, envy being plainly the cause of the complaint. "It made me furious to see those little puppies enjoying something I couldn't have any more!" We have known a feeling of this sort to be experienced also by a man who was watching his wife feeding their child.

The children, who early in life were discontented, and those who were satisfied with the quantity and quality of their food, are plainly discernible through character differences throughout life. Gastric disturbances leave an indelible mark upon the disposition of the individual, and it is clear that a great deal of envy exists connected with the impression that others get a great deal more enjoyment out of life in many ways than they do, apart from food. These patients disagree with the world at large or with their neighbours, in the same way that their food disagrees with them. We will also frequently find that a gastric attack will occur either when they are feeling jealous of somebody or if they have had a quarrel.

It is therefore very much to the interest of the peace, as well as to the future health and happiness of the community at large, that we, as nurses having the care of infants, make the most strenuous exertions to satisfy the oral demands of those who come into our change, and train their mothers how to do likewise. We need to teach them to see that it is a matter of real importance in order to establish psychological as well as bodily health of the child, and not merely a fad of our own, or an advertising stunt on the part of the proprietors of baby-foods.

Long ago it used to be a superstition of midwives and those who looked after babies and sick women that the worry or anxiety of the mother would affect the taste or quality of her milk, so that the baby might refuse it, or being ill-nourished upon it become bad-tempered and fail to thrive. It would also be said that the mother whose breast was refused by her child never forgave it, although she might at times appear to do so or to love this child like the rest. Psychology, and particularly psycho-analysis, endorses these beliefs of ancient wisdom, as it does in many other instances. We will frequently find evidence of this relation between emotional strain or anxiety in the mother and discontent in the infant leading to symptoms of *nerviness*, such as we have already described, as well as the baby's refusal of the mother's breast causing a good deal of unconscious hatred of this child in the mind of the mother.

The Tragedy of Unwanted Children

Such misfortunes occur particularly often in the case of those poor infants who have never been wanted, for one reason or the other. The original impression obtained in infancy grows rather than diminishes as the years advance, often greatly magnified by the subsequent behaviour of the mother, or because she may actually tell the child that it was not welcome. This, it is scarcely necessary perhaps to mention, is always a cruel step to take, even should the mother add that she grew to love the child afterwards; but it is one about which a maternity nurse would do well to warn a mother, if she should confide in her the truth about her negative feelings where this baby is concerned.

It is in ways such as this that a nurse could do so much to help mothers and their children, if only they knew how to make the best use of their opportunities to stress the importance of the mother's attitude towards her children from the first, and just how very much it matters to them to feel that they are loved or not wanted.

Influence of Disappointment in the Sex of a Child

Another injurious influence which often jeopardises a child's subsequent happiness is the disappointment of father or mother over the sex of the hapless infant. The result which constantly follows is that the parents strive to gain their wish by making the child resemble the desired sex as much as possible, sometimes even to the extent of giving the child a name or nickname to create the illusion that they really have got what they wanted, boy or girl as the case may be, while the same tendency appears in the clothing and education. Generally the child is only too ready to fall in with these suggestions. But nevertheless it leads to an unhappy and frustrated life, since the man who wishes to be a woman, or the woman who can never forgive Fate for denying her manhood, can seldom rest content. Sooner or later they develop neurosis as a means of attempting a compromise and to escape from accepting the reality of their own sex, which is abhorrent to them, because of their envy of the other. The manifestations of these wishes are often to be observed in quite young children, and may attract the notice of a nurse, especially if she be acting as matron in a school or children's institution, or as school nurse.

The feminine little boy, as a rule, is neither popular nor happy at school. The rough ways of his companions and the compulsory games usually lead to some illness or accident, which qualifies him for a temporary refuge at least in the sick-room or at home. He will also frequently go sick a few days before school reassembles, so that he cannot return, or a few days afterwards. He may likewise crumple up before examinations, which have an important unconscious significance for these children especially, and once in the sick-room it is difficult to establish convalescence and recovery, which means that the hardships which caused retreat will have once more to be faced. We should remember, however, in this connection, that the child himself is by no means aware of the unconscious process that underlies his breakdown. While in the sick-room he is usually a favourite, and it will be said of him that *he makes such a good patient, and never grumbles about all the happy times he is missing that the other boys can enjoy.* He knows that *he* would not enjoy them in the least, but he is anxious not to let the others know that. He will be tractible and popular with the matron or nurse, of whom he will be very fond, because he usually puts her in the place of his mother, to whom these children are typically devoted, and he will often be made a special pet because of his gentle ways and nice manners.

The masculine little girl more often comes within the sphere of the nurse as the result of accident, through her own foolhardiness, or to prove that she can do the same as her brothers, rather than by illness, especially of nervous origin. She would seldom *crock-up* if she could help it, since her creed and ideal of manliness puts illness outside the pale as a sign of typical feminine weakness, to her way of thinking. She will be inclined to an over-indulgence in games or sport and run the risk of serious physical strain rather than admit any limitation of her own endurance. She will also never own to feeling pain, which may sometimes baffle those who are attending to her after accidents, because they will take what she says literally without considering her ideal which would make her scorn to acknowledge it. Knowing her type, and it is usually plain enough to a discerning observer, it is easy to make the necessary allowance for her scruples, and then follow the line of our own deductions. Later on, having made friends with her by tacit sympathy, since the offer of any other variety would be disastrous, because it would be considered, together with the person who suggested it, *sloppy,* we will be able to discover all we want to know without much further trouble. There will be more to be said about these two types later on, in the chapters devoted to the nervous troubles of men and women respectively, at present we want merely to sketch in the outline of child neurosis and the sources whence it springs.

Results of Oral Deprivation

For the moment we must return to the difficulties of the infant and its first disappointments in life, which mean so much for its subsequent health of mind and body. Still further problems will arise in connection with the all-important subject food-mother-love that it is not surprising to find these components assuming vast proportions in the nervous troubles of adults and children, to which the name of Oral Neuroses has been given. We have already referred in the previous chapter to neurotic trouble as representing a deficiency disease of the mind or the emotions, with love in the central position as the main desire that is felt to be so conspicuously lacking, and which the patient struggles to acquire by all means that can be found. This inordinate need for love, including *the person* (the mother or nurse), in the first place, from whom it is desired, and, in the second, as the proof of her love, *the food*, although something else may take its place later on, may not infrequently be traced to some actual deprivation of this kind during infancy. This may have been the consequence of some illness of the mother, or because a suitable food could not be found for the child to replace the natural one, which was physically or psychologically impossible from the beginning.

For reasons such as these the usual physical advantages of breast-feeding may be strengthened by those that emphasise the psychological benefits, which are both many and momentous. We should especially bear in mind the latter problem relative to breast-feeding. Occasionally the baby, even when breast-fed, may not be satisfied physically nor psychologically because of the poor quality, as well as an insufficiency of milk. In such a case, being put to the breast only provides a constant source of disappointment and a sense of frustration for the infant, who finds that all the efforts in the world cannot produce the blissful feeling of satiety which its little mind and body crave, which may leave behind a queer longing always to get more than it needs, should the opportunity to do so arise, because at some time the supply may fail once more. The deprivation will stamp itself into the child's mind as a culminating possibility of tragedy, to be hungry without being able to satisfy one's hunger, and this feeling of uncertainty may often lay a foundation of mistrust that is never really eradicated, because the child will feel that the mother is deliberately withholding the food. For this same reason we may draw the conclusion that to tease a baby by being late with its feed, or by giving it an empty bottle so that its look of disappointment may amuse us, perhaps to cure it and punish it for greed, is not a method we should recommend, because of the serious consequences that may arise which are not usually taken into consideration.

The children whose early feeding was sufficient and regular, and who suffered no untoward experiences, become confident and trustful that others will fulfil their obligations and promises with the result that their expectations are usually correct. They are, in fact, the people who do not consider the possibility of denial, and so get what they want, often through the effect of the power of suggestion upon other people with whom they come in contact. If they should happen to meet refusal, of course they will be much surprised and frequently exceedingly disappointed. In their turn, however, they will generally be found to have a strong, reliant character, and are equally prepared to carry out their own obligations. It is usually the deprived child who turns out the insatiably greedy one, because of this lurking fear, dependent upon the early trauma, that its wants may at some time not be satisfied in the future; and it will frequently be suspicious of impending injury when it is neither imminent nor intended.

Feeding Sick Children and Adults

It is the common experience of all that food plays an essential part in the nursing of sick children as well as that of adults, and it has already been mentioned as a nursing problem in the previous chapter. With these remarks in mind we will probably remember many cases that will provide illustrative details. We shall also be able to recollect corroborative data that the food interests of the infant are revived in the sick adult, showing itself in antipathies for certain kinds of food or extreme fondness for others. Perhaps we have noticed the frequent preoccupation of the invalid with the topic of food in general, not only concerning those that suit him or her, but also those that do not, or the greediness of some patients who always seem to want something provided specially for the sick-room, and show anxiety lest anyone else should have any that remains after a meal. Then we also know that absolute lack of interest in food shown by others, which may come from the same source as those others, which we have been describing, and serve as a past defence-reaction against future disappointment, typical of the saying, "Blessed are they who expect nothing, for they shall not be disappointed." The child who was bitterly disappointed in early life in any respect will often repress wishes in any way connected with the original disappointment, so as not to suffer a repetition of the acute distress again in its life.

Loss of Appetite

This leads us on to that important subject, loss of Appetite, always a matter of interest to the nurse, and one upon which she is often required to summon the entire resources of her professional skill. Even in the infant we find this symptom occurring should a loved person or the one who usually gives food to the baby be away or unable to do so. The stranger is frequently far from acceptable to the infant at any time, and it does most certainly not want to be fed or handled by one who is unfamiliar or whom it does not like, particularly when ill. Thus grief remains throughout life a typical destroyer of appetite. So also is anger, for the angry person usually refuses to eat or to partake of food with one who has been the cause of the annoyance, and who has prepared the food to be eaten. We remember that we have noticed that the infant regards the food and the provider of it as one, therefore if the one is out of favour neither can the other be received. Moreover, to the child mind, to refuse food is a way to trying to punish the person who brings or prepares it, so that she should have had this trouble in vain, and we will find that this idea exists also in the mind of the person whose food is refused. She is annoyed, just as we have found the mother never forgives the infant who refuses her breast. It is by no means rare to find a sulky older child push dinner away and say he or she does not feel hungry, if table manners have been corrected; and we find that the man who has had a quarrel with his wife will go out to dine at his club, because it seems particularly obnoxious to him to partake of food that the offending person has had anything to do with, such as ordering or preparing. When love is uppermost, then food that the loved person has arranged, cooked, or brought, takes on additional attraction.

Hunger-Strikes in Infancy

The infant who went on Hunger-Strike during weaning, rather than accept a substitute, may often repeat the manœuvre later, once more trying to win a battle against adults by attempting to force their compliance because they are afraid of the consequences if they refuse to let the sick person have his or her own way. Parents are nearly always alarmed by this persistent refusal of food by the child, and usually try all kinds of ways in which to tempt back the appetite, because the child who is not taking its food properly quickly presents a pathetic figure. It must also be remembered, nevertheless, that this child does not look a whit more unhappy than it feels. In the struggle to regain the parents' love, symbolised by their giving in over the food question, it is showing clearly just how much it is needing reassurance at this particular time. Something of an unusual character has probably happened to cause the child to feel that it needs such strong proofs of affection to restore its confidence in its parents, as well as in itself, and to fill up the love-deficiency that is being felt keenly just then. All of these problems require investigation before we can be certain what we should do for the best.

Stammering—An Oral Neurosis

An American psycho-analyst, Dr. Isador Coriat, in his book *Stammering—A Psychoanalytic Interpretation,* is anxious to prove that this disturbance of the speech function in children or adults is an Oral Neurosis, due to an early trauma, which has left its trace in this desire to gain gratification in sucking, biting, or playing with words. He also points out that the baby delights in similar pleasure and in making the same sort of gurgling noises, which many stammerers repeat very frequently before they can make a start, or sometimes, having started, will use to interrupt what they were saying. Other investigators, however, although many agree with Coriat that the psychological elements in the defect far outnumber the physical causes, feel that there are other equally important roots of the trouble. Stammering has been treated successfully by psycho-therapy, including psycho-analysis, although it always ranks among the forms of psychological illness which do not respond easily to treatment of any kind.

THE TRAUMA OF TEETHING. CONVULSIONS AND BREATH-HOLDING

Normal weaning and a consequent change in the diet of the young child usually coincide with teething, an experience that provides a good deal of pain and discomfort in any case, and it will be responsible for a number of other troubles for the baby, as well as for the household in general. The appetite is then almost certain to be a minus quantity, because of the pain in the gums, in addition to which the resentment caused by the change in food will serve to make matters worse. Sleep will also become irregular at this time, for the same causes, however well and soundly the baby has slept before, and disturbance of its bowel habits may join in the general confusion. It is usual nowadays to regard inability to sleep as indicative of psychological or emotional excitement, and it is always a likely occurrence when unfamiliar experiences present themselves before the child, or during pain, grief, and mental agitation. Not only do the adults become somewhat short in patience, when confronted by a wailing, sleepless child, fretting because the teeth are slow in erupting through swollen, throbbing gums, but some children themselves show equal annoyance with their discomfort and appear to imagine the injury to be caused by somebody else, or that it could be relieved if someone took enough trouble to do so.

For this reason we occasionally see the teething child turn and strike the nearest person or itself in anger, but we should also reflect that this muscular discharge is the natural reaction to muscular tension, and at the same time will help to relieve the general psychological tension caused by the continual pain. Another complication commonly associated with both the digestive and teething troubles of infancy is that known as convulsions, and a similar condition, although rather less serious, when the child who has been crying becomes more violent and holds its breath until it is cyanosed and the limbs become rigid. Should we carefully observe when attacks of this kind happen, we often find that they follow closely some occasion when the child cannot do something that it wishes, perhaps because of lack of skill, as well as when somebody has thwarted it in some way.

It may also be caused by fear, some sudden shock, or a bodily injury. Dr. David Forsyth, in a most illuminating paper, "The Rudiments of Character," published in the *Psychoanalytic Review*, April 1921, describes this condition minutely in a footnote to some remarks upon the closely allied disturbance, psychogenic epilepsy. He writes as follows:

> Psychogenic epilepsy thus represents a deep and inveterate unwillingness to face life, even the most elementary, and serves as the fulfilment of that wish which, as was indicated earlier, must be the first wish of every new-born child.

Then as the footnote we find:

> It is only necessary to watch the infant work itself into a fit to realise how completely this explanation meets the facts. As its annoyance grows into overpowering anger, it drops the rattle in its hand (renouncement of the pleasures of the world), turns from the mother or pushes the bottle from its lips (disavowal of alimentary wants), holds its breath until black in the face (repudiation of the lowest function under its control), and finally becoming unconscious (return to the vegetive state), wins the only haven that gives shelter from every vexation.

The child quickly discovers if this method be successful in attracting attention, or if those around become afraid of allowing it to cry in case another attack of breath-holding should be induced, and it will readily take full advantage of this useful method of gaining power over its environment. In many cases, especially in rather older children, the preliminary stages are sufficiently protracted for anyone experienced in baby's ways and not afraid of them to be able to distract the child's attention by arousing some other interest before the attack has had time to develop.

In point of fact it is a common experience of the nurse that the baby, who for any reason has not been allowed to cry, becomes an expert in making use of the threat, and we will find this child prolonging the going-to-cry-in-a-minutes expression in order to give others time to make terms with it if they wish to do so, or warning them of the consequences if they do not give in. Thus it used to be a general belief that little boys who had a congenital hernia, or any tendency to weakness of that kind, must not be allowed to cry or scream, because screaming might at any time produce a rupture. When a mother believed this to be possible and acted upon her belief, she would take precautions not to allow this child to do so. In this way the little boy was thoroughly spoiled, since he always got anything he cried for, while his sister, about whose health the mother entertained no such fears, went without and was allowed to cry as much as she wanted to.

Some mothers have a particular aversion to hearing any child cry, for reasons intimately connected with their own early childhood, and so always capitulate before the threat of tears, with the usual consequences. On the other hand, however, we will sometimes find people with a strange wish to make children cry, and never feel that any scolding has been effectual until it has attained this result.

Should we happen to observe the difference in behaviour of the same children when they are with their own parents, who are amateurs in the art of looking after either the sick or the healthy child, and when a professional nurse is in charge, who has had plenty of experience of difficulties of this kind, our usual deduction will be that the nurse, who is not so readily alarmed by eventualities of this kind, does not find children nearly so prone to try experiments of the sort upon her as they are when she is away and the parents are alone with them. We should also bear in mind that the baby quickly misses the support which is derived from the calm presence of the trained person, and will for this cause be more happy and content in her company. We will also remark the same need in the adult neurotic patient, subject to similar hysterical or anxiety attacks, who will frequently say before the nurse goes off duty: "Please don't go out of the house, because what would become of me if I were to have an attack while you were away? Nobody else would know what to do with me." The fact that the baby as well as the adult knows that someone is at hand who can be relied upon to be able to deal with any emergency, often prevents the necessity for putting the matter to the test. The same influence will affect a nervous horse, when an experienced driver takes up the reins a fresh confidence is brought about.

Training in Cleanliness

It is impossible in this one chapter to deal with these difficulties of childhood in any but the briefest way, and to point out some of the most common danger-zones in the early training of the child which offer vantage-ground for the construction of subsequent psychological disorders. It is usual for all kinds of nervous illness to show regression to an earlier stage of mental or cultural development than that which the patient has achieved, just as physical illness necessitates a similar regression to a state of dependence upon another and a resumption of the habits of childhood. We find this to be also the rule in the food requirements of illness, and it will be equally clearly marked in those other important aspects of infant or adult nursing, those of bladder and bowel function.

Before birth the infant is not voluntarily concerned with either process of elimination of waste matter from the body.

Urine has occasionally been found in the amniotic fluid, showing it to be present before birth, as well as the fact that it can be excreted, although defæcation occurs after birth only. For some considerable time after birth, micturition remains both a reflex and involuntary action, being the result of discharge of the bladder when it becomes unpleasantly full, and the peristaltic action of the bowels regulates the passage of fæces in a similar way at regular intervals in the healthy baby. The modern nurse, taking advantage of the natural mechanical processes of the infant, will try thus to establish regular habits in the baby coincident with early training for cleanliness from the start, and in accordance with the baby's own rhythmic tempo. This is naturally a much wiser course than that of leaving the matter entirely out of consideration until the baby has learnt to derive considerable pleasure from irregular habits and then striving with much vigour to break those already made to so substitute others in their place, which generally means an obstinate struggle between two human beings equally determined to have their own way.

Reactions to Interference

We should realise that some babies develop two things exceedingly early, the first is hatred of interference, and the other a sense of pleasure connected with defæcating in a certain way and when they please. Even quite young children often discover that a greater degree of this pleasurable gratification may be obtained from passing a constipated stool than one which is normal, or by use of a fluctuating movement of the sphincter muscles, half passing it and then withdrawing the fæces again within the anus, which "play" often forms the baby's first attempts at practising self-control.

A great many babies, therefore, at an early age strive hard to maintain their independence in this significant question of bladder and bowel function, and realise their power of control over the urethral and anal sphincters to this end by refusing to obey the wishes of the adults who are anxious to train them to good habits, and continue to urinate or defæcate only when it pleases themselves.

Rudiments of Self-Control

It is interesting to watch the infant gradually gaining control of these muscular actions which at first were entirely automatic, and to notice the uses to which the baby puts this newly acquired power. In these respects the methods of those in charge of the baby will play an important part. Some will try persuasion by love: "If you love me, you will do this to please me!" Others prefer the opposite tactics: "If *you* don't do what *I* want, *I* won't love *you*!" Again, there is the alternative of punishment and fear. "Do what you are told, or you will be sorry for it. I will punish you and give you some nasty medicine!" or, as a last resource to conquer the constipated (obstinate) child, the enema or suppository will be used, which the child consequently regards as a punishment.

All these types of incentive for action, which have been originally connected with excretory functions, will often become the model upon which all subsequent behaviour is constructed, and the struggle for power will assume such large dimensions that these functions will gradually absorb a quite disproportionate share of the child's attention and interest, as they also frequently do in the thoughts of the patients who suffer from hypochondria and some forms of neurasthenia, such as were described in the last chapter.

We may regard these early manifestations of the baby as worthy of our serious attention as nurses, because of their importance in later life, using our understanding of the situation generally to recognise that those responsible for the care of the baby may often be the prime movers in the struggle, because they enjoy mastering it eventually as a gratification of their own desire for power. A great many people can be exceedingly aggressive towards young children and demand their obedience in such a way as to provoke refusal, because consciously or unconsciously they like the battle in order to win in the end, and make the vanquished one own to being beaten. This desire to feel stronger or more efficient than others will frequently be only too apparent in those who have chosen as their life work the charge of the helpless, be they infants or sick adults.

Child's Struggle for Independence

The child who is taught to attend to the function of its bowels for love of the person most closely associated with its care, or to avoid punishment, may in the first instance refuse this love-offering, should a quarrel have taken place between them. According to this pattern, we shall find a period of constipation taking place, concurrent with any emotional experience of later life, in order to punish the loved person by refusing this fundamental sign of love. On the other hand, when punishment has been the result of failure to defæcate, the sense of Guilt is aroused in connection with the process, since to the child's mind punishment essentially follows wrong-doing. Guilt brings shame in its path, and may, as a reaction and defence against both, provoke defiance, with the logical consequence—constipation, because it would rather be punished than give in of its own accord.

We find these children showing the won't-give-in-until-the-last-minute reaction in the general routine of daily life, getting-up, going to bed, and the like. They will put off everything until the eleventh hour, and often wait until another does the thing for them, or makes it imperative for them to start, repeating, in this way, the action of the adult who finally forced their resistance with a strong aperient or an enema. We can thus see that this is not a good precedent to establish, and it finally causes the adult in charge more trouble than if they had exercised increased patience in the first place, to teach the child regularity of habits, through observing its own rhythmical tempo, and training it in accordance with that, than without regard for the child's natural process of peristalsis, to suit their own convenience.

Results of Childish Habits in Subsequent Illness

These early tendencies will be reproduced in exaggerated forms during nervous troubles, both those which occur during childhood as well as in mature life, for this habit of procrastination and inability to act upon their own initiative is typical of neurotic patients. All actions then become the result of suggestion on the part of another, or of contra-suggestion (the opposite of the direct suggestion), which is going to produce difficulties for the nurse, because the old scenes of childhood will be repeated over and over again, with all the old manifestations of love and hate, guilt and defiance. A short survey of patients who have been in our care will be sufficient to verify these statements relative to the interest shown by nerve cases in their constipation, the action of the bowels generally, and the use of aperients and enemata. Again, in this connection, it is only right to call attention to the other side of the picture and observe the anxiety of some nurses and most hospitals and institutions, unless the mark denoting a daily movement of the bowels can be duly recorded. The nurse in charge of these patients often reacts with a similar show of guilt, and seems to feel that her professional competency will be called in question if those she is nursing have failed in this respect, becoming strangely agitated upon occasions should the time come for her to go off duty with this still unachieved.

The hysteric patient may still treat the bowel function

as a sign of affection requiring a corresponding meed of praise from the nurse, withholding the function in cases of emotional disturbance. We shall see the neurasthenic as inert in this respect as in others, and the obsessional patient making use of elaborate rituals connected with these bowel functions. Those in whom anal sadistic hate is predominant will use this means of showing defiance against the authorities of the sick-room, as in the past the rebellion was directed against those who superintended the early training in the nursery.

Regressions of Illness

Many of these difficulties which we have been describing will appear to complicate the nursing of children suffering from other illnesses as well as from the early forms of neurosis.

For this reason, as well as for many others, the nurse in general practice requires to understand what they may denote, so that she may act with her eyes open and pick up hints from these signs concerning what is going on in her patients' minds, beyond the information gained from other symptoms and the words of our little patients. All forms of illness show the regressive tendency, and just as we notice that the same old feeding troubles of babyhood reappear during sickness, the same abnormalities of excretory function are equally likely to be revived. The child, during the regression to an earlier stage in this lapse from good health, keeps pace all round with the degree of the illness and the regression, which shows itself, on the one hand, in the resumption of a milk diet and the use of a feeding-cup or spoon, and on the other through all stages of bowel irregularity and uncertain cleanliness, which since were surmounted, until the condition of incontinence and involuntary action of the bowels is reached in the course of the illness. This recognised symptom that denotes the weakness of the patient marks also the degree of seriousness reached by the morbid invasion of the personality shown in the temporary destruction of standards which have already been reached.

Before we can accurately gauge the amount of regression, and consequently the divergence from physical or mental health that has taken place, this cultural standard must be ascertained, especially in children, although it is useful to know what it was in childhood in the case of adults also. In the instance of children brought up in homes where habits of cleanliness are extremely rudimentary or casual, incontinence would probably occur at a much earlier stage of illness than among those who had been brought up very strictly in this respect. Equally an adult will not so readily become incontinent as the child, because the control of the excretory functions is a habit which has been longer established, and therefore takes longer to break down than one which has been more recently acquired. We always find that in cases of illness, fatigue, shock, loss of control of any function takes place in this order, the last to be acquired is the first to disappear, until we are left with the most rudimentary instincts and reflexes.

It is by no means uncommon to find that the symptom of incontinence on the part of the patient provokes a negative reaction on the part of the nurse. For this subject especially she seems to lose grip of her professional knowledge that it is a symptom, and one that denotes severe illness, and not merely a recurrence of *childish naughtiness* on the part of her patients, young or old, which must be *punished* in some way so that they will exert more self-control. This attitude will usually be the reaction of the young nurse who is very positive and anxious to save herself as much trouble as possible, it is true; but it is amazing to observe how often it will occur in those whom we should have thought would have not allowed their personal feelings to swamp their professional obligations and the knowledge they have acquired, yet in this we may also see a clear instance of last to come, first to go, in respect to acquired knowledge cutting across old teaching of childhood.

We have already pointed out that among children as well as adults in whom this subject was connected with extreme guilt and humiliation in childhood, this condition of incontinence during illness will reanimate similar feelings of shame in the past. Matters are made worse should it arouse comparable feelings also in the nurse, in addition to which we find disgust and contempt of the patient for the lack of self-control. Her feelings will quite certainly by some indication, even should they not be expressed in words, be communicated to the patients. This nurse's attitude naturally enough reflects difficulties and experiences of her own early training, which taught her to regard such lapses from good habits of cleanliness as utterly reprehensible, from which she has constructed the opinion that a lack of self-control is the most despicable of all human failings, and that it is a thing apart from the signs and symptoms of bodily illness. Nurses often seem to hesitate from accepting all the changes that are concomitants of illness, including these as well as emotional fluctuations.

It is a frequent impression that we gain from nurses that it is the apparent lack of self-control on the part of neurotic patients which provokes their dislike. Should we examine this trait of the nurse in the light of the foregoing remarks, we may see that it is more than likely that the exaggerated value placed upon the possession of self-control by herself, in contrast with the lack of it in her patients, often accompanied with a total lack of sympathy, if not of open contempt, for those persons in whom it is not so highly developed, comes from just such a source in the first instance.

Results of Incontinence upon Character

Unless this symptom of illness has been handled wisely we may find serious results in the character of the child, and it will often happen that a period of involuntary action of the bowels, when habits of cleanliness have been already established, will frequently be the collapse of self-confidence, especially should the child have taken considerable pride in the former acquisition of self-control. It has been a surprise of a very unpleasant character, as well as a shock, to find that this control can no longer be exerted, and that a return to baby ways must be made *nolens volens*.

In nursing children through a serious illness, when this is bound to occur, we as nurses should be careful not to add to the child's feelings of guilt and humiliation by words or actions of our own, because of the unfortunate results. We know that muscular control cannot be maintained concurrently with extreme physical weakness, and we should do our utmost to help the child over this additional misfortune of illness, with all the understanding and sympathy at our command. We have to lead the child back to self-control of this kind as physical strength returns, just as we have often to teach those who have been seriously ill once again the use of legs to walk and run with, which to the active child may equally come as a shock and blow to its pride in achievement.

Concurrent Neurosis and Physical Illness

A great many early expressions of psychological trouble in children seldom come into the professional nurse's care as such, but only concurrently with physical illness. The early cases of hysteria, obsessional or anxiety neuroses, that are unfortunately only too plentiful, rarely gain recognition for what they are, which naturally precludes any form of adequate treatment. Those who have an hysterical tendency will be termed naughty or highly strung. When they are obsessional they will be called peculiar, with odd little tricks or habits. But they may be taken to a doctor and nursed on account of symptoms arising from conversion hysteria. Once again they may be left to grow out of the trouble, or relegated to some educational backwater, if they are already showing signs of dementia præcox, and thought of as backward or lazy. This, by rights, should scarcely be placed with the neuroses, since it is a condition that when fully developed is usually grouped among the recognised forms of juvenile insanities, although the distinction between some of the psychogenic and mental illnesses is difficult to formulate, except from the point of degree of severity and of divergence from the standard of accepted normality.

Children Suffering from Hysteria

The child who suffers from hysteria differs in little from the adult troubled with the same complaint, except that the child's variation from standard child behaviour is not so wide as that of the adult, who in the course of the illness falls back into signs of child-behaviour. The desire for love, to attract attention as well as the wish for excitement, opposed to a hatred of monotony, are the same as in the adult. The struggle to gain some advantage over rivals is in no respect changed, except that in childhood we will see it in its first stage of direct manifestation, with this setting actually in the home, and the *dramatis personæ* will be the father, mother, brothers, and sisters, should the child not be the only one. This, however, will frequently be the case.

The young hysteric is often the victim of the Œdipus Conflict, about which so much has already been written that it will scarcely need much explanation here. The child tries to come between the parents and capture the love of one or the other exclusively, generally that of the parent of the opposite sex, whilst doing its best to vanquish or exclude the rival. Illness will frequently give the otherwise helpless little one a better opportunity to attain these wishes than when in health, and so advantage will be taken of the least indisposition to magnify it as much as possible and make of it a vehicle for the fulfilments of wishes. Very often, moreover, in the case of the little girl who has hysterical attacks, the aim is the same as that of the little boy—to refuse to be pacified by anyone but the mother. We shall then find that the signal for their occurrence will be that the mother has a party downstairs, and so will be forced to leave her guests to attend to the needs of the child, or that the father is wanting her particularly. The hysterical little boy, on the other hand, often appeals to the sympathy of the father as well as that of the mother.

We should remember, nevertheless, that hysteria may appear in the symptoms of physical illness only, and consider this possibility when engaged upon the nursing of young children, especially after we have made careful observation of the home conditions and compared the child's normal position in the family with the results obtained by illness. When we have made careful observations and have come to the conclusion that the symptoms are partly due to emotional difficulties in the child, we shall realise that the situation presents additional problems than if we had physical illness only to nurse. The combination of the two will be the more complicated to cure, and the illness takes on a more serious character because of the hysterical origin rather than being of less importance, which might be a popular belief.

Let us discuss the question and try to see why this should be the case.

The first step is to recognise the fact that we have now one illness complicated by a second, which increases its severity rather than cancelling it; that the origin of the trouble is thus made the more obscure than if it rested upon the physical basis alone, and that it may be difficult to remove the child from sources of reinfection, even if we cure the present attack, just as though we were to nurse a child through enteric and leave it in a highly infected area, full of typhoid carriers. A future such as this would certainly cause a nurse to feel anxious about the fate of her patient, even after a temporary good recovery.

The first step is difficult because the tradition has not yet been abolished that teaches that hysteria is nothing and that the neurotic complication cancels the illness rather than increases it. A general understanding of nervous disease is not yet reached, which makes the *absence* of realisation of this increase impossible, since we may still read conflicting statements such as the following in a textbook for nurses. The section from which the paragraph is taken is headed *Hysteria*, and the paragraph itself, *Nursing*. These are the actual words:

> If it is, however, wrong to sympathise, it is equally wrong to let the patient see that *you know there is nothing the matter with her*, as that will result in losing her confidence, and with it the chance of doing her good.

The italics are those of the writer of the present book. Can we truthfully say, "*we know there is nothing the matter with her*," when we have already admitted that she is suffering from hysteria? This is a direct contradiction, and it is remarkable that a medical man cares to place a statement of the sort in a textbook written for nurses studying during their training, since it is far from representing the most up-to-date information at present available among members of the medical profession.

In these psycho-neuroses which provide so much difficulty for the nurse and so many complications of the physical symptoms that may be present, the chief concern, as in many of the physical diseases, is to discover the source of the infection or the malady. This must be found before the course of the trouble can either be checked or recurrence prevented with any certainty. When found, what is the next task? This also lies along the same lines as if we were dealing with an external infection. To remove the cause, or to immunise the patient from further infection by building up a strong resistance, will be the two courses open to us. In the case of emotional disorders in childhood we are faced with considerable difficulty when we attempt to remove the cause of the psychological infection, neither is it an easy matter to immunise the patient from further infection. The chief reason why this is more difficult in childhood is because the child is actually living in the danger-zone, the home, among the people who may be causing the damage all the time, and that the risk of reinfection is consequently ever-present. When we come to nurse adult psycho-neurosis the origins of the disorder are lying far away in the past, and have been recalled from memory through a present event which is similar, the adult is really far more free to deal with difficulties even in a present situation than the child, who has no say at all in the management of affairs and frequently has only the route of illness as a method of escape from an unbearable position. Freud long ago pointed out that the hysteric patient "suffers for the most part from reminiscences"; with the adult in his mind, of course, we should remember, however, that the child hysteric is labouring under the burden of present unhappy events, such as the adult patient finds oppressive in retrospect.

Cure of the Hysteric Child

As we have already said, we must arrest the disease and prevent recurrence by abolishing the source of further infection or by immunising the patient. How can this be done in cases of hysteria and other forms of neurosis? What are the sources of infection, as well as the predisposing causes of the complaint? How may we discover them? and when discovered, what can we do about them, either in the matter of removal or by strengthening the resistance of our patient? For these tasks become a matter of grave responsibility to the nurse.

We may try to avoid our responsibility by saying that after all this part is a question of diagnosis, and therefore should rest with the medical man in whose charge our patient is. But duly considered, the nurse might have a far better opportunity to do this than the doctor who sees comparatively so little of the patient, and especially of the child in relation to the rest of the family, which often gives us the clue that we are seeking. Also, we should remember that the parents, as well as the child, would probably be inclined to talk more freely to the nurse and before her than in the presence of the doctor. She can, moreover, observe the child's behaviour when in the company of the parents, as well as their attitude towards the child, even should they not be together in the home, but only visiting for a short space of time during the visiting-hour of a hospital.

The cause of the child's neurosis is usually something that forms part of the integral home relationship, and it is hard to change it for this reason. In the first place, the parents may not consider it the place of the nurse to suggest any alteration in the parental treatment of the child, so she may have to try to exert her influence with the doctor to get him to put the new point of view to the parents. Secondly, so many people frequently play a part in the formation of the neurosis that it is sometimes difficult to change the attitude of all of them towards the child, even were the parents inclined to be ready to take our advice and help us in carrying it out.

Still, this same battle has been fought in the past in respect to feeding and open-air improvements that have been made in the care of infants and young children, when it was considered essential for the child's health that changes of the sort were to be made, and therefore, when the nurse sees that this other aspect is equally important, it will help her to take the right course to bring it about likewise. She will be better equipped for the conversion of the parents should she really understand the roots of the difficulty and the tendencies in the parents which are causing the trouble from their side. If she can convincingly show them that it will conduce to their own comfort and peace of mind, as well as an improvement in the health of the child, she will find her task considerably lightened. The neurotic child is certainly as grave a problem in the home in many ways as the one who is a cripple or suffering from any other bodily infirmity. Once more we would like to point out to the nurse that she needs to be a leader of public opinion in this important matter of treatment of psychological disorders.

We have already hinted that some difficulty in the home itself may have been the cause of the neurotic illness or of the development of some slight indisposition into a serious illness. What may some of these danger-points be to which the child with a predisposition to nervous trouble will fall a victim?

Predisposing Causes of Child Neuroses shown with Physical Signs

First among these may be mentioned absence of the parents or a nurse, when the illness serves the purpose of recalling this beloved person to look after the sick child. Second, may be ranked the advent of a little brother or sister, who has apparently alienated the affection that the little patient used to feel all his or her own. The idea of separation, whether actual or metaphorical, causes a lowered vitality. The child becomes intensely unhappy, and thus the physical resistance to illness is lowered so that any possible infection in the environment, or that which is already in the child's system, claims our little patient.

The best-loved person may then return to nurse the ailing child, in this way restoring what is most desired, which may quickly re-establish health. But, on the other hand, it *may* prolong the illness, because the little one may fear that once he or she is better the mother or nurse will go away or return to the care of the rival. It should be avoided, if possible, that a child has to encounter too sudden or severe deprivations in its early life, when it is in health, so that it can only gain attention and the signs of affection when it be ill, since this puts an altogether too high premium upon sickness to be salutary for a child with any tendency to delicacy of any sort, and may easily be used to gain what is so urgently needed.

Regression to the state of illness may also occur should the child be confronted by a psychological demand for advance mentally or physically, perhaps emotionally, that is to behave in a too grown-up manner, which is altogether beyond its powers, and dreading failure will fall back upon a diminished attainment which is well known and familiar, so that no difficulties can be experienced and there is no chance of failure.

What happens in a case of this sort when a professional nurse is called in? It may spell either grave dissatisfaction for a child who greatly dislikes substitutes or bring supreme content. The former is the result for the child who is wanting *the real loved person*, the latter when the child is looking for *an ideal mother* who will lavish more attention and love than the original person has bestowed. The nurse and patient between them arrive at a happy transference situation, and the child accepts for the time being a new mother in place of the one who is felt to have abandoned him or her in the hour of need, and cure will be established through identification and the wish to give this kind mother the joy of bringing back the child to health, which often becomes a rebirth phantasy.

Consequences of the Transference Situation

The consequences of the transference situation and the way it is handled afterwards will lie in the hands of the nurse, and speak for the amount she knows about her own psychology, as well as that of the child she is nursing. By means of the transference and the influence of her own disposition, through identification, as well as her conscious attitude to life, she may be able to build up the little one's nervous health at the same time as that of the body, because of the facility with which the child always copies anyone who is loved and who loves it in return. The nurse, nevertheless, should be on her guard against a too great love on her side of being first and remaining first in the affections of her patients. The sick child must eventually be given back to the parents and not permanently stolen away through the transference, so that he or she will continue a chronic or recurrent invalid, through the presence of a nurse having become an emotional essential to happiness, so that the little invalid wants to have the sole attention of one person and to be the recipient always of her kind ministrations.

This is just where the nurse must know herself very thoroughly and watch her reactions carefully, should she find that her little patients show any tendency to cling too long and tenderly to her, or to make slow recoveries with long convalescent periods. In some cases her part will also include acting the part of an extremely tactful mediator between the child and the parents, but of course without the knowledge of the former. She may be able at some time in the course of conversation to give them a few hints about the care of emotional health, their own as well as that of the child. In a good many instances she will also find it necessary to show them a new appreciation of their own child, and to lead the way to the inauguration of a fresh standard of home proportions. It will be noticed that this course of action is exactly what was suggested that the nurse should carefully avoid in the case of the adult patient. This alteration in attitude is one of the chief differences between the nursing of the child and the adult, and rests upon the psychological differences shown in the actual presence of the child's difficulties and the large part played by phantasy and memory in those of the adult.

Nervous Exhaustion in the Child

It frequently happens that the nervously disposed child who falls ill is one whose vitality may have been exhausted through exceedingly strong, energetic, and capable parents, who, having always been vigorous themselves, do not take into consideration that the physique of a child cannot accomplish everything that is easy for an adult. This may sound ridiculous on the surface, but it happens so frequently that one feels justified in calling attention to it. The child's limit of endurance cannot compete with that of an adult, apart from its courage, which may try to do so either in walking, games, or keeping its attention fixed upon any one occupation for a long time. The parents, likewise, frequently do not realise the difference between the adult and the *child mind*, as well as body, and are apt in consequence to feel that the child gives in too soon, and has not enough pluck or even ability to make a more determined and protracted effort, when this is far from being a just estimation of the true state of affairs. It may be that the parents certainly do not express their feelings in words or even acknowledge it to themselves, but children will quickly be aware of their disappointment and may exert a physical strain to keep going longer than is good for them, so as to counteract their parents' poor opinion of their powers of endurance. When this still fails to have the right effect, we will often see them flag and know they are feeling miserable at being unable to come up to this impossible standard, which, of course, the child will never realise is beyond its age and strength.

An Advantage of Physical Illness

The child who has been definitely declared ill is no longer expected to make efforts henceforward, because the illness and not its courage will be considered the cause of the disability. Therefore we will often see a child who is ordered a long rest appear relieved and become restless when the end of this reprieve draws near, which means that the efforts will have to be resumed. We shall have to try to rectify this difficulty of anxious expectation concerning the termination of illness, as we should also have to do if we were to notice too much gratified importance being derived from the illness. Ill-health should never be considered a goal of ambition, nor should it become associated with humiliation and shame in the mind of the child, frequently an echo of parental strength that despises weakness. Out of our abounding health and strength we should be merciful, but not patronisingly so; considerate of the young and weak, yet not emphasising too much the inevitable disparity between adult superiority and childish inferiority or helplessness.

The Race to Catch Up

This struggle to keep up or to catch up may also take place between ambitious youngsters and the elder brothers and sisters. All these causes of psychogenic trouble we have mentioned should be considered among the origins of children's neuroses, or physical conditions of ill-health that have been aggravated by emotional strain. The nurse has such excellent opportunities of listening to the ideas and opinions of her young patient that she will thus gain a shrewd notion of the cause of his or her difficulties, without the child being aware that things of importance are being communicated. In her answers she may often be able to straighten out perplexities for the confused child, through giving explanations about these differences of accomplishment due to disparity in age, through showing that it is quite natural and in no way anything to be ashamed of, as well as a condition that will certainly mend itself in time. In numberless little ways she can thus help the worried child, once she has gained his or her confidence, remembering always the very great therapeutic value of putting troubles and grievances into words, whether the patient be young or old. Spoken about and looked at carefully with the help of another sympathetic person, many troubles lose their sting and may be readjusted with a little thought and care.

Home-Sickness. A Psychological Ailment

The nurse in charge of the school sanatorium or the matron of a smaller boarding-school will come across a good many difficulties of this kind among young children, and hear from them about their troubles at home and at school. She will also have excellent opportunities to observe the various complicated physical conditions that arise from the emotional strain called *home-sickness*, caused by the separation of an emotionally unbalanced child from a parent, who will frequently be equally disturbed by the loss of the child. In some cases we will discover that this child has been in the habit of sleeping with the mother, often, indeed, of sharing the same bed, and that in going to school the first break has been made in this custom. Under these conditions the separation, should it be accomplished without too much distress, which causes the psychological breakdown of either, will be of inestimable value for mother and child, because the former close union was the evidence of a far from healthy emotional fixation which would lead to grave trouble when separation in due course became a necessity. The transference to the nurse in these cases especially forms a useful bridge leading from the old weakening bond to a new and more healthy relationship to the mother, as well as a psychological splint to the fractured affections, until reunion can take place with better adjustment and greater freedom of movement for the child as an independent person, no longer overwhelmingly relying upon the parent.

Functions of the Nurse in Recovery

In a similar way a child's illness in a hospital may make a salutary loosening of the too close tie of home, and strengthen the growing independence of the child. We must, however, be prepared for the over-affectionate parent who has encouraged the dependence of the son or daughter, accusing us of undermining home influence and coming between them. But then, strangely enough, we may often find blame instead of thanks for restoring a child to nervous *health*, when the ideal of the parent has preferred a *lass with a delicate air*, or a fragile, ethereal little boy. We are bound to run the risk of difficulties of this kind when we try to do our best to build up the health of children from this angle, and are obliged to add to our primary nursing activities by trying to readjust the ideals of the parents into more robust and sensible channels.

Another very real function for the nurse in playing her part in the illness of children is to track down and allay their fears. Some of these arise from what they have seen or heard concerning the illness of others. Many will be derived from an over-active imagination, books, or from that very important cause of fear, the Unknown—all of which become greatly exaggerated in cases of anxiety neurosis. This often makes a vantage-point of the fear of illness itself, and a belief that such and such a disease is undermining the constitution, because some symptoms may be felt which are known to exist, from hearing about them in connection with a friend or relative. Again, there is another matter for us to ponder. As nurses, we have become so familiar with the idea of illness and even of death that in this way it has become shorn of the fear that many lay-folk will feel in connection with both of these eventualities. We may even reach a stage when we forget entirely that others, whom we come across as patients, are still very much afraid of all its strange rites and ceremonies. For some, the sheer unfamiliarity of illness presents considerable uneasiness, especially the unusual experiences of the hospital ward, while the operating theatre, and perhaps a death in the next bed, will certainly be an immense shock to a child who has never come in contact with death before at such close quarters, if at all, and we should be prepared to try to alleviate it as much as we can.

A frightened child is often helped by the fact that a grown-up person takes the trouble to try to find out what is the matter, should this not be obvious, and then does not laugh but sets to work to try and allay the fear with some explanation of the circumstances that are troubling the child. We often find that a simple explanation of what is going to happen when the first preparations for an operation begin, and that it is not going to be carried out then and there, including what it will be expected to do when the time comes, proves a great relief of anxiety to a nervous child. So many children find that if they are allowed an opportunity to think things over and do not have to come to them suddenly and unprepared, they are able to get through a strain of this kind without nearly so much difficulty as having to face the shock of meeting the Unknown without any mental adjustment. This feeling is equally prevalent in adults who have not had much or any experience of illness of any kind. They are longing to know what is going to happen, and what will be expected from them, so that we shall discover that they will be most grateful for a few hints from the nurse concerning the routine about to be experienced for the first time.

One of the most necessary warnings in the nursing of sick children is to remember never to deceive a child. We often hear people going out of their way to tell a child emphatically that it is not going to be hurt, or that nothing is going to be done, *the doctor is only going to look*, when they know quite well that some painful treatment is going to be carried out, or a minor operation performed without an anæsthetic. They say that this causes the child less worry and cuts out sad anticipation. But from experience we find that the child usually most bitterly resents having been duped thus, and in addition will become suspicious in the future and believe that no one can be trusted. A large number of fears that appear in children past infancy, which cannot be accounted for otherwise, have been subsequently traced to an occurrence of this nature, or to some minor operation carried out during infancy without an anæsthetic. It seems to be a fairly general medical belief that the young infant does not feel pain, and that consequently many operations, such as circumcision especially, may be performed without an anæsthetic. The baby's cries and struggles to free itself are taken as merely the result of reflex action and need not be considered as of any importance, since all memory will be effaced as soon as the actual stimulus is over.

Psychological evidence, however, shows the contrary to be the case, and that these old painful memories linger on in the background of the mind—the Unconscious, from whence they reappear at a later period, showing themselves as fear of pain and of men and women, especially of being held tightly without the possibility of escape; while a haunting dread remains that the very people from whom one usually expects love and protection are the very ones who are aiding and abetting this cruel torture. A feeling in the child generally corroborated by the fact that one or both of the parents or the nurse held the baby while the doctor performed the operation.

This brief outline of the origins of child neurosis will give the nurse an idea of the state of affairs existing in the mind of the child, whose sick body she is striving to cure and restore to health. The troubles of the adolescent of both sexes and their difficulties to adjust to the new conditions of dawning maturity will be referred to later in the two following chapters on "Psychogenic Troubles Prevalent in Women," and "Psychological Disorders Common among Men and Boys." We find that in a great many essentials they will recapitulate the neurotic conditions of childhood, while they take on a fresh colour as well as a bolder outline from the changes effected by time and environment, which commonly means a shifting of the scene from the original limits of the home into a rather wider field of school life, which implies new transferences to teachers and schoolfellows, often in conflict with those original bonds that still cling tightly or loosely, as the case may be, between parents and children.

ÆTIOLOGY OF PSYCHOLOGICAL DISORDER AND EMOTIONAL CONDITIONS IN CHILDHOOD

Prenatal Influences

Suspected of being of great importance, but evidence indefinite at present, since the material at hand cannot always be corroborated by actual facts of the case.

Birth

This trauma in the life of the infant probably exerts much influence over the child's future and its attitude towards life and death. Freud states that this forms the origin of *anxiety*. Regression shows in many forms, including that of convulsions, psychogenic epilepsy, and dementia præcox, a desire to resume the undisturbed bliss of uterine existence.

Early Environment and Training

Difficulties arising at this period will furnish origins for general nervousness, restlessness, and irritability, as well as many of the other more definite forms of neurosis found in children.

Disappointment of the Parents connected with the Birth or Sex of the Child

Child feels that it is not wanted or loved. It becomes dissatisfied with its own sex and envies the opposite, striving its utmost to become as near this as possible.

Weaning

Difficulties at this stage often lead to all forms of Oral Neurosis, gastro-intestinal symptoms, hysteria, anxiety, and convulsions.

Training in Cleanliness

This not carried out wisely provides many of the anal-erotic and urethral neuroses, as well as some of the symptoms of neurasthenia and the obsessional neuroses.

Attitude of Parents to Child: too much or too little Love

Leads to the formation of the familiar forms of neurosis connected with the Œdipus Conflict, hysteria, etc.

Advent of Brothers and Sisters

Increases any neurotic tendency already existing in the child, who will often try to rival the elder ones, causing physical strain, or the effort appears to rival a favourite baby through illness.

Separation from the Parents

Regression in face of difficulty leads in many cases to increase of physical illness to recall parents or to concentrate home attention upon an invalid. Dependence upon the parents or revolt against them leads to defiance and adoption of a parent substitute, in doctor or nurse, who is welcomed through illness.

Adolescence

Dawning maturity and recapitulation of childhood with repeated physical tendency to renewal of illness or neurosis. Physical strain of puberty. Renewal of transference situations.

BOOKS WHICH MAY BE READ IN CONJUNCTION WITH THIS CHAPTER

1909. *Children in Health and Disease,* by David Forsyth, M.D., D.Sc., F.R.C.P.

1924. *Das Trauma der Geburt,* by Dr. Otto Rank.

1924. *Love in Children and Its Aberrations,* by Oskar Pfister.

1928. *Stammering: A Psychoanalytic Interpretation,* by Dr. Isador Coriat.

1928. *The Unconscious in Action,* by Barbara Low, B.A.

1928. *Difficulties in Child Development,* by Mary Chadwick, S.R.N.

1929. *Psychology of the Infant,* by Dr. Siegfried Bernfeld. Translated by Rosetta Hurwitz.

1929. *Nursery Life 300 Years Ago,* Edited and Translated by Lucy Crump.

1931. *Simpson,* by Edward Sackville-West.

CHAPTER V

PSYCHOGENIC TROUBLES PREVALENT IN WOMEN

In surveying psychogenic troubles, or their particular forms, which are supposed to be more general among women, we should remember that some of the characteristics that are regarded as neurotic symptoms, when they appear in an adult developed to such a degree as to interfere with the normal functions of life, are instilled into the little girl at an early age as part of her necessary training. It is true that this greater severity respecting the nursery education of the daughter, in comparison with the relative freedom from restraint of the son, has relaxed somewhat of recent years, but it is still to be met in many families even at the present day, and we constantly find its reverberations among adult patients suffering from neurosis, whom we have an opportunity to observe.

Among these survivals we may especially notice a fear of talking to or before strangers, of travelling or living alone, and anything which in nursery parlance might be considered *not nice* or *rude*. Again, we will find many of these same persons with a rooted objection to hearing about a new idea or taking up any fresh work which had not been familiar in their old home. When these women were young, they were certainly taught that little girls were to be seen but not heard, and that, like Red Riding-Hood of old, it was dangerous for women to go about by themselves, or to live by themselves. Since that time these warnings or prohibitions have grown so great in their minds that in many instances they have swamped the reality of changed conditions, so that the old injunctions are still carried out literally, or the situation is so much feared that the life of the persons will be considerably crippled where use and pleasure are concerned. Furthermore, the psychological symptom will in addition serve the purpose of adding or taking away something which makes the dreaded action or event impossible.

In the case of one girl who suffered from violent pains in her back, they would make it impossible for her to continue a walk or dull shopping expedition that was in progress with some other person, sometimes even a visit to a museum or a strange locality. The pain would usually be more intense when she was accompanying another person, whose pace was rather greater than her own, or when the project did not offer any very great attraction to herself. This pain in her back was convenient in many ways, all of which were originally unrecognised by herself as benefits, although she was well aware that there was some unwanted element in each of the situations which were thus prevented. For instance, to walk far was a matter of dislike, for two reasons at least, one being that since childhood she had an unconscious fear of being lost. When quite a small child she had either lost herself or had fancied she had done so in a garden skirting a large wood. The unconscious fear argued as follows: if you went a long way from home you were more likely to be lost than if you stayed in the near neighbourhood, therefore the conscious reaction to correspond with the fear was to immediately get into some vehicle and make for home as soon as the pain came on. The other important reason connected with the various occasions when this pain made itself conspicuous, besides that caused by the fear of being lost, was urgent need to go to a lavatory, and not knowing where to go because one was in a strange place or out of doors—an anxiety state caused the pain. To ask her way in a shop was for her quite unthinkable, and the fear of needing to relieve herself when it was not convenient for her to do so caused the most intense feelings of shame and anxiety.

False modesty of this description concerning the bodily functions appears in many disguises among the neuroses of women. Especially in this matter of urination do we find that the little girl has been more strictly brought up than her brother. She will, therefore, consider it one of her chief feminine disabilities, which consequently places it also in the first rank among her dissatisfactions with her own and her envy of the opposite sex. We may equally reckon this as one of the most notable results of the strict early training of the little girl, since it commonly originates from over-emphasis placed upon modesty.

Traditionally, it seems to have been taken for granted that all women were inclined to be hysterical at times simply because they were women. Upon rare occasions in the past, when physicians put forward the suggestion that men could also be found who suffered from symptoms identical with those considered typical of the female hysteric, they were received with derision by their colleagues, although the opinion is admitted without comment to-day.

The original cause that was ascribed to this derangement of emotional balance was a displacement of the uterus, and a reference to this condition, containing the earliest known forms of cure, was quoted at length at the end of the first chapter of this book. In their observations of this malady the ancients, however, were partially right, although the origins to which they traced the symptoms were often incorrect. They knew that many women become periodically unbalanced, emotionally and mentally, but they mistakenly connected these changes with wanderings of the uterus about the woman's body on the one hand, and with the phases of the moon on the other, rather than with the cycle of her menstruation, which, like the moon, recurs at a period of twenty-eight days. We are now beginning to recognise more clearly how closely a woman's delicate adjustment of psychogenic balance fluctuates in accordance with this periodicity. But we will return to this subject later in the chapter.

For the most part the nurse only comes in contact with the woman who suffers from a psychological disorder when it is already extensively limiting her normal life, or when it exists concurrently with some other which she has been called in to attend. The various symptoms seem at first incomprehensible and irrational, and only take their place in the picture when we realise their possible origins and the important part each factor played in childhood, rather than in the present adult stage. The neurotic person, of whatever actual age, usually continues to regard the world at large and the people of her environment from the child's point of view, and to some extent will continue to reason as a child and retain a child's lack of proportion respecting the relative importance of various functions of life.

Let us partly re-examine the ground covered in Chapter II in order to bring it into focus with some further details and types of women's neuroses, showing their relationships one to another as far as possible, and to ascertain what forms are most commonly met with in certain temperaments or at different ages.

Hysteria may well serve as our starting-point, not only because of its historical associations, but since the symptoms which appear in the adult hysteric coincide in so many ways with those we may observe in any infant who is emotionally upset, or when suffering from some passing physical disorder. They have one great difference, however. It is thought that the adult suffers so acutely from such small apparent cause, because the present-day trifling stimulus recalls some very serious psychological trauma of early childhood. "The hysteric patient suffers for the most part from reminiscence," Freud tells us in his first book (*Studien über Hysterie*). When we are dealing with the psychogenic conditions of childhood, we have actually the wounds themselves before us, and not merely their scars, which are represented by the neurotic symptoms of adult life.

We may say with truth that a child can show the symptoms of hysteria at any age, although the term is not often applied to the emotional disturbances of young children or infants. The typical symptoms will be present nevertheless: sudden excitement, laughter or tears, sometimes following one another with extraordinary rapidity or overlapping; anxiety, breathlessness, palpitations, difficulty in swallowing, sudden defæcation, micturition or vomiting without adequate physical cause, except that the organs of the body join in with the disturbance of the mind. If we observe the adult hysterical attack it will remind us of the tantrums of the baby, or its sudden outbursts of inconsolable grief. It is as fruitless in the instance of the adult, as of the infant, to appeal to any standard of logical reasoning in our attempts to check it when in progress. Still, we should observe in both instances the exact circumstances or persons that contribute to its occurrence, as well as the actual result which is achieved through its agency. These two factors may be considered as influential among the contributory causes of its appearance, and will provide some valuable information concerning the best methods of preventing recurrence or dealing with the situation if and when it should be repeated in the future.

Let us summarise briefly the predisposing causes of hysteria in the child, because when we come to examine the history of the adult in detail we shall not infrequently notice an early outbreak of the same kind in childhood. We have already described Hysteria as a *psychological deficiency disease.* The little hysteric is essentially a child for whose happiness and emotional welfare much love and the outspoken protection of the adults is required. They are notably easily influenced little girls, readily malleable through their affections, a tendency of which others may take unwise advantage. They need love and happiness so much that they will often impulsively surrender much in order to keep the love of others, and in addition work hard to win the approbation of those around. They also require constant reassurances of love and tenderness, but will be equally generous in giving them in return. We shall find them very sensitive to any rebuff to their often too lavish display of affection, which will usually provoke their tears that sometimes will have the result of softening the hearts of those about them, so as to restore their attention and pity.

The exaggerated emotional fluctuations of the hysterical persons are nearly always detrimental to the plans of the household, and we usually find that the latter must undergo complete revision before they can adjust themselves to her requirements. By this means the hysteric child, man or woman, achieved a great deal of power in the home, sometimes through the hysterical attack itself, at others by the threat of its imminence or possibility. The patient is usually very quick to estimate the power that can be gained in this way, as well as to learn accurately to discriminate between those persons who will be easily influenced by the symptoms and those upon whom they make very little impression.

The hysteric wants to be first in love, in attention, or in illness. She appeals to the unconscious elements and wishes of others by a pseudo-flattering petition for something that cannot be gained from another, since no other person is so nice or so kindly understanding. This appeal, originally made in childhood to one of the parents, will be now repeated to the nurse during the illness of an adult, and is aimed at the nurse's unconscious wishes, connected with either her scarcely appreciated or her conscious estimation of herself, which forms one of her greatest difficulties in nursing such persons. It is generally directed at the nurse's most vulnerable point, the most significant joint in her psychological armour, and should it achieve success through giving her patient what she wants, she will then be used as a pawn in the game of the neurosis, which will make the possibility of a cure uncertain. For this reason it is essential that we know in what ways, and to gain what sort of attention, these appeals will be made, as well as the kind of tendencies in ourselves that will respond to such pleading; for few of us are entirely unshakable, provided that we are asked for something which gives us some pleasure to bestow, or which, in some fashion, proves us to be the sort of person we would like to be thought.

The picture we sketch of ourselves in the sanctum of our own minds, and which we often spend our entire lives in trying to substantiate, plays a greater part than we often realise in our vocation as a nurse. We want to be a mother to the weak and a strong protector to the helpless, to gain our power through the love of our patients by making them fear and obey us, or to advance ourselves in the sight of authorities through our professional skill. Therefore, in order to gain one of these wishes, we play the part of the kind mother, the stern mother, or the learned mother; but the hysteric has a corresponding form of appeal for each, something that each one exclusively may supply, and by so doing appear pre-eminent in exactly the way we desire.

Neither does the hysteric only desire love. In a curiously distorted fashion some of these patients like to feel themselves hurt by those they love, and wish to be scolded by them, scorned by them, or treated roughly and harshly. By means of these requirements their appeal can find equal favour in the eyes of the severe type of nurse, who is often recommended because she is considered *so good* for the patient. But she encourages the neurosis, rather than freeing the patient from it, so that she may be left independent and not continually in need of a stern mentor at hand to dictate suitable behaviour.

It is thus a doubtful *good*, because it offers such an intense gratification to the *masochism*, as it is called, of these patients, and increases rather than diminishes their dependence upon another human being. They wish to be dominated and treated severely by the nurse, because of the thrill they gain from it. This situation will most probably be a revival of nursery scenes of childish naughtiness, which took place then to provoke punishment, or even whippings, from the mother or nurse. It was excitement that was welcome, and a mark of attention in any case from the beloved person, and as such to be desired.

In this connection it is interesting to note the reactions of the female hysteric to the male doctor, and to observe his response. We should remember that the emotional little girl was not always exclusively attached to her mother, and she made use of the hysterical attack sometimes as an appeal for paternal as well as maternal protection. The child who wanted the mother only represents but the one type, that of the mother-fixated child. The hysteric, however, is as frequently the little girl who was making very persistent attempts to capture her father's love and to rival her mother, whom she might simultaneously inconvenience by the same means—the attack. The child who sought her father's attention or protection will certainly strive to win some special marks of preference from her medical adviser. She will make use of similar subtle appeals to his sympathy or chivalry, his wider understanding or wisdom, which will be all very flattering to the psychological ideal he has of himself as a physician, who cherishes the thought that no one has a better understanding or influence upon nervous cases than himself. This will be particularly plain in his attitude also to the nurse, who represents the hypothetical mother, to whom, unconsciously, the boy, now grown to man's estate, may frequently harbour an ancient grudge, which might cause him to take the part of a pseudo daughter, the patient, when she appealed to him to champion her against this substitute mother.

Where we find this inordinate craving for love, we may frequently notice a group of supplementary tendencies, which give rise to heightened neurotic tension—namely, Fear, Anxiety, and Guilt. The principal derivative of these symptoms, which may cause the nurse considerable difficulty, is Jealousy, that shows us grave mental complications, such as *distortion of reality*, by means of which the patient will refuse to accept signs that another is preferred, and on the other hand to manufacture proofs where none exist, save in her own mind, to corroborate a wish. Both of these conditions are extremely frequent in the forms of neurosis that are associated with jealousy. Together with this constellation, fear, guilt, jealousy, we will notice many of the familiar symptoms of the anxiety hysterias or anxiety neuroses, and by further transitional steps where other factors blend we arrive at the obsessional neuroses, paranoia, melancholia, and the manic depressive states. These offer prominent difficulties for the nurse, as well as much interest, since they show the various ways in which the patient may try to circumvent abhorrent truths that love is not for her but another, and the evidence of failure to gain what is longed for.

Fear commonly springs up in the life of the child when it feels alone and helpless. It has been summed up briefly by Freud in the infant's realisation of the absent mother, as portraying the lack of all that is essential to life and content. The infant for whom this sense of helplessness is the most unbearable soon develops different means of finding ways of recalling the mother or of preventing her absence. By this means it creates a barrier or defence, which prevents it coming face to face with the dreaded situation. We may thus find that many fears of children are subsidiary, and present some difficulty, or offer some excuse, to make the presence of the protector, the mother, absolutely indispensable, so that the child will not ever find itself alone.

This element of wanting the mother appears directly in many types of both anxiety hysteria and anxiety neurosis. The child who is afraid of the spider in the room, or of the dark, is immediately pacified if the mother comes into the room and stops with the child, although she may not succeed in catching and expelling the spider. The adult suffers from some forms of anxiety so acute that it becomes necessary for somebody always to be present for fear of what the patient might do in a panic. The patient gives this impression to others, or is herself convinced that she is not safe without the presence of another, this other person usually being the mother herself or the nurse who will represent her, and who, it is felt, can protect her from any calamity that may arise : an attack of breathlessness, sudden blindness, or death itself.

The patient is sometimes afraid to go out alone, to be in an open space or a closely confined one, but the fear abates if another person is there also, which arouses our suspicion that in many cases the symptom exists in order to have a plausible excuse to gain company and sympathy for something that will be better understood, like a fear, rather than the vague feeling which might be called loneliness, that possibly might only call forth ridicule. In retaining the person of the much-desired mother, the child feels that her love is assured. It also serves the purpose of preventing this person from devoting too much time or attention to a rival, in which case we shall find the addition of a jealousy factor. If she is present, we know what she is doing, and that she is not with another.

This state of affairs often complicates the duties of a nurse in charge of several patients. For instance, on one occasion a nurse on night-duty was put into a position of great difficulty by having three patients in a ward of some twenty-four cases who made use of this fear factor to claim her attention whenever she was engaged with one of the others. When she was giving some special treatment to one, another of the three always had an anxiety attack, which seemed to the patient a justifiable claim upon the nurse's presence for a few moments at least, and naturally this made it necessary for her to leave what she was doing at the moment. One of these patients suffered from acute heart trouble with attacks of dyspnœa, which stimulated intense anxiety or vice versa. Another was an elderly person who was expecting to undergo a serious operation on the following day, and wanted reassurance of the nurse to help allay an extreme fear of death. The third was a patient suffering from dysentery, who always called to her for assistance relative to this trouble directly she had been hurried to the bedside of one of the other two.

The presence of the anxiety consistently gives its possessors a belief that someone must come to the rescue, or it may be used as a defence against unpleasantness by establishing a truce with the dangerous person, instead of the barrier or fear which has already been described. Thus the plea, "I am afraid," may serve to divert the attention of the person away from something the child has done, or turn it in another direction in order to reassure the child that the thing feared cannot possibly be. In both cases it serves the purpose of a child in that it may transform anger into sympathy. This manœuvre will often be seen in the child in relation to the two parents, and we shall find it recalling a fear when one parent is about to scold itself or to caress another, thus concentrating the attention of all concerned upon the one who is frightened. A great many children will suffer from fear because it has been suggested to them by the quite well-intentioned but mistaken questions of an adult to a child who is crying: "What is the matter? What are you crying for? Are you afraid of something?"

The playing-off of one parent against another we have

already mentioned as being repeated in the behaviour of the patient in respect of the nurse, the doctor, or some male relative. When in the original situation the motive of fear was to claim the mother from the other brothers and sisters, perhaps even from the father, the patient will show more concern to gain the interest of the nurse, through her fear, in competition with other persons in the house, or in rivalry with other patients in the ward or nursing-home, so as not to be left alone, or to retain her services altogether in private practice because she feels that no one else would understand her so well.

But in many cases of anxiety hysteria we frequently find that the little girl, by means of her fear, seeks to win her father as chief protector, or to enlist his sympathy against those whom she feels are molesting her in some way. As a repetition of this impulse we find the patient seeking an opportunity to hint to the doctor that the nurse is not so attentive as she might be, or is not carrying out his instructions. By this means she may try to remove the nurse and at the same time to flatter the doctor by showing him that he has her greater confidence and gratitude. We shall also notice that some patients always want their doctor sent for, or at least to know where he is, should they feel than an anxiety attack is approaching. Sometimes nothing short of his visit will allay the fear, but in other cases to learn that he is available if necessary, has been informed, or has sent her a message that she can take a dose of his special medicine, often acts as efficaciously as the charm of an ancient medicine man.

It is natural that the woman hysteric who needs her doctor to be the chief person in her cure will be inclined to show the negative side of her reactions to the nurse, and will not be inclined to carry out her orders, nor to be much influenced by her words. The nurse, representing the mother of the old nursery situation, will be unconsciously, if not consciously, regarded as the rival-in-chief; and the nurse, if not aware of what is going on in the patient's mind, and why this state of affairs should be taking place, may resent it and feel offended that the doctors should always be appealed to in a crisis, and her own reassurances are of no avail. In point of fact the nurse may often become jealous of the influence of the doctor in these particular cases, especially if she have a tendency to this emotion arising from her own childhood, when perhaps a brother, or her own father, always seemed to be referred to in a dispute rather than herself, and she is still unable satisfactorily to separate the events of the present from those of the past.

The patient, it should be remembered, is not acquainted consciously with the actual motive that lies behind the fear, and without doubt suffers acutely from these anxiety attacks. Any sign from those present that the patient is "putting them on" or pretending, hoping by this means to check them, usually increases rather than diminishes them as an attempt to convince all present, including the patient herself, that it is a real situation. The experienced fear is real enough, but its accent is frequently misplaced upon the screening fear, rather than the far more dreaded possibility which lies beyond, which is too terrible even to contemplate.

When we come to consider the various ways in which women deal with the dreaded situation *Deprivation of Love*, which is the second stage representing the lost person, what other morbid conditions may we find arising from this situation, and in what ways may the nurse in charge of such a case be involved in technical perplexities, as well as in actual difficulties, that concern her relations with the patient and others of the household?

A great many apparently physical illnesses which punctuate the life of the nervous or neurotic woman form what may be regarded as appeals for love, tenderness, or care. They will often take place when some loved person is away, so that it will be necessary for him or her to be recalled; or should the attention of this person be thought to be waning, thus causing a diminution in attention, the illness may serve the purpose of an attempt to bring back the attention to its former focus, and deflecting it from another person. We may also find that this will occur should another person in the house be ill and needing considerable care. The desire to be the most ill person will have quite disastrous results, although at the same time the hysteric may bewail the fact that she could not have chosen a worse time to be laid up, when there is so much to do. There is a great deal to do, it is true, but naturally a sick person cannot be expected to do anything about it, and so others have to see to the whole business until all the invalids are better. An illness, it should be remembered, always effects a truce.

These illnesses, which so frequently punctuate the life of neurotic women or men, are often of pyschological origin, and are known as *Conversion Hysteria*. In them we find a condition that has been called *Organ Speech*. We may observe that a part of the body will in some way, often through loss of function, represent an idea or wish that cannot otherwise be put into words. In some cases it will act as a defence against an idea, or an action on the part of the self or another, in the same way as the *fear*, which forms a barrier of protection in the anxiety hysteria. Among the various forms that conversion hysteria may take we may count such symptoms as psychogenic deafness or blindness, all of which will make it impossible for persons suffering from these symptoms to continue to live their ordinary life. Certain occupations or functions of life become impossible because of these disabilities, and it becomes necessary to obtain help from another in order to carry on, or it is necessary to become readjusted to a very limited or restricted life for the future, so that the condition furnished by the fear may be accommodated.

As a subdivision of conversion hysteria we may mention that group of neurotic troubles similar to those just described, which of late years have gained considerable attention from research carried out under the investigations of the National Institute of Industrial Psychology. These are called *Occupational Neuroses*. An important factor in the cure of these rests upon the question of compensation for disablement, and the possibility of pension should the injury become permanent. In such cases the symptom will generally occur after an accident, or it may take place following a period of extra strain caused by a rush of continual overtime work. The symptom differs with the occupation of the patient, but is always intimately connected with it. It will likewise be such as to make the further continuance of the work impossible. For instance, a typist may suffer from cramp when using the typewriter, or a machinist will have neuritis, which makes the use of one or both hands out of the question. The cook has to leave the kitchen because the heat of the fire or the smell of cooking gives her a headache; the children's nurse becomes deaf so that she can no longer hear what the children say; or the musician is obliged to put aside her instrument and take to teaching instead, as "rheumatism" has stiffened her fingers, so as to make her execution inadequate for instrumental work.

In each of these cases the apparent physical disability acts as organ speech, and declares that the person can no longer continue the struggle of carrying out that particular form of work. It records the fact that a change is needed, or a long holiday. Occasionally the difficulty lies not in the work itself, but in the economic conditions of the home, and the disability proclaims a belief that it is time that someone else contributed to the upkeep of the home instead of the entire burden being on the shoulders of the patient. None of these ideas would have been easy to put into words, neither, perhaps, could they have gained this definite result as surely through this method of illness. But there is another important advantage in addition the patient would never have tried to free herself had she been obliged to fight her battle consciously. She would have felt that she was shirking her burden, and would have been ashamed not to have gone on to the bitter end. It is just because of this reason, she had been forcing herself on against the grain, that her unconscious mind had found a way of escape which her conscious mind would never have accepted. For such a person, illness provides the only justifiable reason for putting down tools, or of admitting that she needed a rest from her labours.

It is now apparently the disability rather than her personal reluctance to continue that says "No!" so emphatically to continuing in the same dull and monotonous groove, which in all probability has never offered any great interest for this person, but was the only means of earning a livelihood that offered itself. Change of work, additional interest in the daily occupation, or a recreation for the leisure hours will often effect a cure without medical treatment, or even the massage or electrical treatment that is so often ordered for such cases. This will often be found, nevertheless, to have a most beneficial effect, and through suggestion brings about the cure of such patients, in which we may see the influence of the transference and the result of the patient feeling that someone else is interested in her and is trying to help her.

Better still will it be to show the patient, if possible, an alternative method of dealing with her difficulty at a conscious level, and get her to look at the problem from all sides. She may then try to find out what is the unpopular element in her work, and whether this cannot be rectified in some way short of breaking down, or changing it for another occupation. The cause of the trouble will often be found to be some association with a childish memory, which being revived may sometimes disentangle from the present situation; but in many cases change of work, or removal from an uncongenial environment, may be necessary. The cause of the illness may also be traced to some trouble that has arisen between the patient and some persons connected with the work from whom she wishes to get away, as frequently as it comes from dislike of the work itself. It is much more satisfactory, from many points of view, to deal with our problems of our own conscious accord than to wait for our unconscious to help us out of the difficulty with illness, or as sometimes happens even with unconsciously planned suicide, which has the appearance of an accident.

We may often trace this desperate way out of life's troubles in the strange accidents that occur, which seem as though they could have been prevented. Should we have any intimate knowledge of the hardships of the victim, and realise the struggle that has been going on previously, we often realise the significance of the action that has brought about the attempt at escape.

Another way in which a neurotic patient may try to deal with the problem of loss of love, or disappointments in life or people, is by a mental distortion of the facts and a refusal to believe the evidence of reality. We may find this occur chiefly in two ways. The patient may firmly refuse to believe that she is not a much-loved, popular, beautiful, and clever person, remaining blind to all proofs of the contrary, because the truth would be too painful to be faced, partly because the change to anything more attractive would not be entertained as feasible. On the other hand, should the truth slowly penetrate, the Ego might love itself as it is too much to acknowledge that this could be true, and think that it was the result of the envy or jealousy of those others, because it would be quite incompatible with this type of Ego self-love to acknowledge itself to be in the wrong.

The *Doubting Mania* that is to be found in many cases of obsessional neurosis, and which we have already referred to in a previous chapter, may be considered as another attempt to solve the problems: Am I loved, or am I not? Do I love, or do I hate? In order not to accept the reality of another being preferred, doubt springs up as a defence against accepting the unpalatable truth. I am not loved as much as that other, but I do not want to believe it, and I will not, or cannot change to become more like them in order to be more liked. In these types of emotional illness that strive against reality and realisation of the unpleasant facts of life we usually find a very great amount of self-love and self-admiration. This may be a primary condition, existing from infancy, and fed by the superabundant love and admiration which surrounded these children. They received all homage as their right, and merely wondered and felt peevish when it was not forthcoming, which aroused some such thought as this, What is the matter with these people that *they* do not respond to my charms as usual? The young folks who suffer from early forms of dementia præcox will be discovered with similar phantasies of importance and grandeur, and try to escape from reality to this pleasant phantasy world, which is altered to conform with the child's paramount wishes. A secondary phase of self-love may arise from keen disappointment felt on account of the withdrawal of love by a well-beloved person. The patient feels she may rely only upon herself, and then loves herself instead, as in childhood this mother or nurse had cared for her.

We find yet another type of person who takes a great deal of care to distort reality to suit strange beliefs and wishes. This is the woman who tries to find evidence that she is unpopular and unwanted, often believing that others are jealous of her and despise her, which ideas have a rather different motive as their foundation. If we feel that everyone is jealous of us, it follows that we must also believe that we have much to give them cause for their envy. We feel that we are superior to them in some way. On the contrary, should all despise us, we must have given them cause for this contempt, and must be the most degraded of mortals, therefore inferior. In many cases of this sort, should anyone attempt to offer overtures of friendliness, such patients will usually refuse the invitation curtly, being firmly convinced that it is the outcome of patronage or pity. People of this type tend towards Obsessional Neurosis, where we find delusions of all kinds that are persistently retained in spite of all our efforts to prove them mistaken.

These persons in childhood often believed themselves unwanted, frequently not without cause. They noticed that other children in the family were preferred to themselves, and hated them accordingly, becoming intensely jealous of them. This is yet another of the varieties of the disguises in which deprivation of love may appear, the jealousy that is felt towards the rival is turned round into the belief that the rival is jealous instead, which shows the intention to retain the first place, since it is the defeated opponent who is jealous and not the victor as a rule. The once-loved person, who has failed in some way to come up to expectations, will be violently hated, but this may also after a time undergo the same transposition, and appear as hatred directed against the patient, in the same way as the jealousy has also been changed round, and the woman will feel herself persecuted and in danger from these same people, whom she believes are seeking to injure her or to destroy her plans.

This state is known as *Paranoia Persecutoria*, and offers peculiar difficulties for the nurses who come in contact with these patients, for reasons which we will explain. We have before us an intense craving for love, the fear that it is now all expended upon others, and that although the patient may have once been a favourite, love has now been diverted through mischance, the beloved person has become tired of her, or because jealous rivals have contrived the separation. Suspicions arise that other people, or even the beloved person herself, may be plotting injury on a large scale, persecuting her in some way, that others are accusing her of wrong-doing, although she feels that she is innocent and they are guilty, or that everyone recognises her and talks of her misdeeds wherever she goes. This is the characteristic form in which the Guilt, which is a main trend of this psycho-neurosis, appears distorted, and projected from the self into the world around. The same phantasy may be traced back to childhood, when the patient tells us her history; but it is difficult to know exactly whether this child did develop paranoic symptoms early, which certainly does happen sometimes, or whether she is now looking back into her childhood and seeing there the same distortions of which she is aware at the present day, although she did not regard these incidents in that light when they first occurred. In those days, of course, we will hear that it was the parents, or the brothers and sisters, who behaved badly to her because they disliked her, or were jealous of her. It was they who were unjust, and punished her without cause. Had they only given her time to explain, she could have done so, and shown them that it was not her fault, but that of another, for which she was made to suffer. She could never see that she had been in the wrong or could have made a mistake, and the distortion persists throughout. The hatred that the patient has felt but repressed throughout her life is now finding its way to the surface in the neurosis, and will often vent itself upon the nurse in an attempt at readjustment and revenge. It is well to remember when we are listening to these sad histories that some of the situations should be reversed to gain a true account of what really happened, and not become a too ardent partisan, in case more be expected of us than we are likely to be able or willing to carry out. We may then find ourselves becoming yet another disappointment, and so a fresh object of hatred and a supposed persecutor.

We usually find that the person who was originally the most loved, or whose love was chiefly desired, becomes the object of the keenest hatred, and that the paranoic patient generally found her greatest attraction in the parent of the same sex, for which reason the paranoic woman finds herself in difficulties through her fervent friendships with other women. This condition is extremely common in a minor degree among those who are approaching middle age, although it will be noticeable among younger folks occasionally as a perpetual grievance, with a tendency always to shift the blame upon another. Later in life it reaches outward expression with such vehemence that it becomes a menace to society as well as to the mental balance of the patient herself, particularly in the years preceding the menopause, when the woman begins to suffer more acutely in various ways from love deprivation.

Men also may be troubled with the same distressing condition, but are more likely to be suspicious of the attentions paid by other men to their wives, and believe that they are unfaithful to them. They will equally imagine that they have committed some crime, or are accused of doing so, for which they are wanted by the police, if not by some secret society, whose rules they have broken. Should they be under medical care either at home or in some institution, it will be the male doctor rather than any woman, be she doctor or nurse, who will come under their suspicion of doing them an injury, for the same reason that the paranoic man as a child was frequently attracted by his father rather than by his mother; and we may often find that the boy's father was nervously abnormal in some way.

The nurse will have to be especially cautious in her handling of all patients with even a slight tendency to paranoia, which is easily detected from the conversation of these women, and their eager attempts to enlist our sympathy for their unkind treatment by others. If we allow ourselves to be installed in the position of the loved person, we run the serious risk of not being able to live up to the requirements of our patients, which usually comprise the following somewhat arduous conditions: that we return the love that they lavish upon us, that we show no interest in anyone else, and require the company of the patient exclusively, although we are not allowed to make any demands upon the patient in return. The position will be seen at once to be untenable, and is bound to come to an unpleasant termination sooner or later, which rings up the curtain for the next phase of imagined contempt, neglect, unkindness, suspicion, and veiled hatred. The patient may believe that she is being poisoned, ill-treated, or influenced in some occult way by the nurse, to whom only a short time previously she was so devotedly attached.

These patients are usually responsible for the strange tales that are circulated from time to time of grotesquely bad treatment at the hands of nurses in hospitals or nursing-homes, which gain a certain amount of credence before they are recognised for what they are—the inventions of a disordered brain. The more acute the case, however, the safer it will be to be concerned with the nursing of it, because then all in anyway connected with the case will clearly recognise the true state of affairs. But in slight cases of paranoia, which are often not immediately diagnosed as such, or should the nurse be unaware of the special difficulties that await her, the most intense worry, or even serious mischief, may be caused in a widespread circle, because the patient may not content herself with talking to those around her, but proceed to write incriminating letters, or may go to the police with accusations about her persecution.

When still in its early stages, this disorder may be cured by various forms of psycho-therapy in skilled hands, but unless it is attempted early the outlook is not favourable. Preferably, the patient should be in the hands of a male doctor, about whom the patient has known nothing before, so that he cannot be supposed so readily to have "heard all about her" from others. The nurse herself should not attempt any treatment for reasons we have already explained, yet should be ready with her co-operation and sympathy, believing in the value of psycho-therapy for this type of trouble, since the nurse who considers this form of treatment nonsense usually manages to convey this opinion to her patients, with results that certainly do not have the effect of shortening the cure, even if it should eventually take place.

Frequently these patients seem to suggest that they might be cured by some form of Occupation Therapy, or by giving them some social work, so that they might transfer a little of the interest that is now concentrated upon themselves to others. But in practice this will not be found a successful attempt to deal with the problem. In the first instance it is difficult to find the exact occupation that appeals to them, because the work they wish for will generally need to be done for a person to gain her approbation or love, rather than for the sake of the interest of the work alone. Likewise, to put these people to social work which involves co-operation with others is to invite trouble of all sorts, should the paranoic tendency break loose in the situation of the work itself, which is only too likely to happen. It is true that they will often tell us that they long for something upon which to concentrate their energies; they want to feel of some use in the world; that they are sure there is some work waiting for them which they alone could do, if only it could be found. We may be cheered by these remarks, and set to work to try and find them what they appear to want, or to suggest some society that would be glad of their help. Then we meet with a sudden check, and may be disappointed if we are not prepared for the plan not being a success. One employment that is suggested is too easy, another is too difficult. They feel they would never be able to learn how to do it, and that it would take such a long time. Perhaps they do not feel that what we have suggested is important enough, and that anyone else could do it just as well. This is probably quite true, since these patients may not have any special training nor ability, and certainly are not as a rule anxious to spend much time or trouble in learning how to do anything well. They are more inclined to believe that someday it will be discovered that they have a natural talent for something that needs but little practice to bring it to perfection. They have told us at the commencement of our search for an occupation for them that anything would be better than nothing, but when it comes to the point of making a decision, we find that this is by no means the case. It will generally have to be a very special something to be done for a particular person before it will produce real gratification. Neither does it always follow that the person who makes this complaint really has nothing to do which others might consider her legitimate duties connected with her home or relations, but which, nevertheless, she is determined to have nothing at all to do with. She has no occupation which she wants, nor can she do things for the person for whom she wishes to work. This is usually the more accurate statement of affairs. Frequently, however, she is not aware herself of the thing nor of the person she is seeking so impatiently.

Another phase of difficulty frequently arises between the paranoic patient and the person to whom she is devoting her time and energy, or to whom she wishes to offer her services: it seems to be her most urgent necessity that another should be dependent upon her in some way, and she will not rest until she has made herself indispensable. When she has brought it about that somebody relies upon her considerably, she begins to feel that it is an irksome burden too great to be borne. In many cases the urgency of the first desire has the force of an obsession. Its main objective, to add to her own power and diminish the independence of her victim, for whom she appears to believe she is sacrificing herself to an enormous extent, suggests the old belief in the function of the vampire. Should her victim, however, resist and refuse to become dependent, she is annoyed, and imagines a score of fantastic reasons for the protest rather than the actual and obvious one that many people are unwilling to be under a great obligation to one who is sometimes little more than a stranger, and who, in addition, seldom allows anything to be done for herself in return. Concurrently with this striving to do things for certain other people, we commonly find this marked repugnance to receive little services. They are usually refused ungraciously, because they will be felt to detract from the sense of power that is so ardently desired. Should she ever feel under an obligation, she hastens to repay it instantly, so that she may always remain the creditor rather than the debtor. As we have already remarked, she is probably unaware of what she is actually striving for so ardently, and the desire will only be made clear to her through the careful observation of results obtained through watching the repetition of the series of events we have described, supplemented by the psychological investigation of her unconscious mind and its impulses, which act as the dynamic for her behaviour.

This exclusive and finally fluctuating love for another that is typical of a patient suffering from paranoia has a definite streak of cruelty in it. This may be recognised in the vehemence with which they kiss their victim, flinging an arm around her neck, and pressing so tightly that real pain will be caused. This type of affection seeks retaliation for each fancied lapse of attention from the loved person, and may be said to be a merciless love, wanting to hurt and to be hurt in the course of the love relationship. The features of these people, as well as their facial expression, will commonly portray a certain amount of cruelty and aggression, which has arisen from the repression of their natural outlets of love as well as their deprivation of affection in childhood. Following out the reversal theme, which has already been shown to be prevalent among those suffering with paranoia, we would usually not be far astray were we to reverse the persecution phantasies that are imagined so profusely to be carried out by others upon themselves, and consider them in the light of reversal phantasies of revenge to be practised by themselves upon their adversaries, who were once love-objects. Yet it is rare to find them in this original form.

One further neurotic condition, which we may regard as a product of deprivation of love, remains to be discussed. This is *Melancholia* or *Depression.* In this case the patient admits the loss of the beloved object as well as the love itself, and settles down to readjust life to a pattern of continual bereavement, for which it is impossible to find consolation or compensation. In extreme cases the condition overreaches the borderline of neurosis and becomes insanity. The patient finds admittance to one of our mental hospitals or a similar institution, and is described as suffering from manic-depressive insanity or cyclothymia. She takes no further interest in the affairs of daily life around her, nor in her personal welfare, cleanliness, and food. She sits and stares before her, silent, or perhaps reiterating a few sentences that touch upon her troubles.

The nurse in general practice does not usually come in

contact with patients so deeply afflicted as this advanced case we have just been describing. The protracted silence, the constant brooding, the long periods devoted to tears or religious exercises, make it difficult for the nurse to know what to do for the best. Obviously, if only it were possible, the most satisfactory thing would be to turn the patient's attention to something else; but when the grief is severe, any attempt to do so appears an impertinence in the eyes of the patient. This being the case, we may sometimes be successful by means of an indirect expedient. The nurse may occupy herself with some new and attractive handwork, which occasionally will attract the patient's attention and stimulate a desire to copy it. Any suggestion of this sort would, of course, be complied with by the nurse, since the interest of the novelty would tend to lessen the grief for a time at least.

The nurse will have to be prepared to remain an indefatigable listener to all the troubles of her patient, because of the relief their recital may afford. The treatment and cure of this form of neurosis present a difficult problem, since it is frequently found in an acute form in women who are past middle age, when they are not so accessible to psychological treatment to effect cure as when they are younger, although from the point of view of providing relief of nervous tension it is worth while as a palliative. The various other remedies which are customarily advised, such as change of air or scene, do not have any lasting effect, because the patient still takes her grief and melancholy with her wherever she goes. In many cases, indeed, she would feel guilty of the greatest negligence if she were to forget her troubles.

The element Guilt plays a very important part in this disorder, for which reason we frequently find that it becomes associated with religious mania. The patient strives to find absolution from her sins through religious exercises, and with the fervour of ancient penitents, who sought to atone for their misdeeds as well as to find relief from their melancholy through the scourge and the hair-shirt. Unfortunately, the true melancholics rarely succeed in finding any permanent consolation in this flight to religion, or it would more often establish their cure. The guilt being duly atoned for, peace and comfort should be found, as well as the still more important factor of the liberation of the patient from the bondage of the past, because a new spiritual love-object would be put in the place of the old one, through which replacement a satisfactory compensation would be accomplished.

At the present day we may observe a most interesting attempt to regain the love-object which has been separated by death in the revival of spiritualism, by which means contact with the loved one will be established through the services of a medium, automatic-writing, or some approximate system. These substitutes certainly can and do often provide great comfort for those who believe that in this way they may actually communicate with those whom they once loved and now have lost. But one cannot help feeling that these people are easily satisfied when reading an account of the messages that are supposed to have been received. Still, we should keep in mind that a very small dose of comfort sometimes comes as a great relief to a very sick soul, especially should it be a direct wish fulfilment, and that this comfort so derived partakes actually of the nature of hallucinatory gratification, a condition in which the desired phantasy supplements or replaces reality, such as we see in the insane who are happy in their delusions.

The magnitude of the guilt that is common in these depressive conditions has a rather curious source. It arises partly from the guilt originally impressed upon the young child in connection with the idea that its wrong-doing has forfeited love, so that the loved person has been taken away. Sometimes, in point of fact, the definite threat has been made by a parent, "If you are so naughty, I will go away, or I will send you away." Occasionally the isolating agent will be represented as God, He will send someone away, or will not love the child any more on account of its misdeeds. This old menace will provide part of the guilt that is felt, but a considerable portion has been transferred to the patient in order to save the loved person from being thought unkind or unjust.

The child in the past was faced with a conflicting problem of this description. It feels that one or the other of the parents has acted wrongly, but at the same time loves him or her so dearly that it is more painful to feel this dear one can have acted thus than to suffer the guilt itself, for which reason the child believes itself to be mistaken, and that it is in the wrong, so introjecting the guilt and seeking to atone for it in some form of self-punishment. It seems far better under these circumstances to bear the double share of guilt and to be able to continue to believe the dear one blameless than to struggle to keep love unchanged in spite of recognising parental injustice. This being the case, paranoia and melancholia present us with two opposite mechanisms, because, whereas the personal guilt in paranoia becomes projected from the self upon others, the patient suffering from melancholia or depression introjects the guilt of another, and seeks to atone for this wrongdoing through endless grief under the guise of mourning for the lost love-object. At the same time, nevertheless, the self-reproach present may hide the kernel of a very rudimentary condemnation of the loved person before the repression was established, which prohibited admitting the loved one had been unkind or unjust, and from this angle may be a punishment for the sin of criticism of the parent, which is not consciously recognised.

In connection with these forms of psycho-neurosis we

will often find a sense of failure predominating in the mind of the patient, which may even have a fatalistic tinge. Some person or circumstances over which the patient herself had no control whatever is supposed to be the cause of the perpetual lack of success. Among these depressive conditions we may frequently find some tendency to suicide, which represents one or more wishes, namely, to escape from life and all its burdens; to rejoin the beloved person, should death have been the cause of the separation, or we may sometimes find the motive of the suicide is to make the person sorry who caused the disappointment in the first place, as well as other still more complicated ideas.

The sense of fatality which may thus haunt life is in itself the greatest possible hindrance to success, since the belief that all attempts are doomed to failure will preclude a wholehearted striving after success. Again, a very deep unconscious fear connected with the idea of success may lie buried in the minds of these patients, which suggests that it may involve some penalty, which will often be responsible for a halt being made within sight of success, or cause a breakdown when some signal conquest has been achieved. The trouble will sometimes depend upon the revival of a gratification of some very old and much desired wish, or suicide may even take place under similar conditions. In one case of this kind the cause was traced to the mother of a patient having told her, as a child, that she might do as she wished, but she would find that it would only lead to unhappiness. The child had elected to have her own way, and the mother had been careful to point out that the result did not bring the child any particular joy, which had set the stamp of fatality upon the realisation of wishes for her for life.

We may observe an attempt to escape from predestined adversity in those persons who fervently adopt the creed of reincarnation, finding therein a solution of the difficulty by a hope for compensation in the future. One of the chief tenets of this belief we will find of especial interest in connection with the woman's idea that she is doomed to failure, which is the comfort they derive from the theory that in their next existence they may change their sex. This deeply rooted dissatisfaction with their own sex will repeatedly disclose itself as the fundamental conception of failure, and the reason why, because of being a woman, no success can be reached. "If only things were different" is a phrase heard perpetually upon their lips, applied to any event of daily life, although arising from this major disability, which has dogged their steps from childhood onwards, although, perhaps, it may be said to create the greatest amount of havoc where marriage or its possibility is concerned.

When this discontent first appears in childhood varies according to the different experiences of each child, but it is rare to find a girl who shows no trace of it at all during her early years. The views of those responsible for her upbringing, and the influence upon her life effected by the presence or absence of brothers, will be seen in its proportions as well as the actual results that shape her later life. The nodal point at which we see it obviously becoming a grave menace to the developing girl is naturally at adolescence, when the onset of menstruation shows her the woman has essentially different functions from those of the man. Here she reaches a distinct parting of the ways, and we will find that this may be reckoned the third of the critical stages in the life of the woman, this dawn of her maturity; the other two being Birth and Childhood, during which, of course, she must often upon many occasions have come to grips with her wish for masculinity.

Those nurses who come in contact with girls at adolescence know what a large percentage go through a period of loss of nervous balance at this time, when one or more neurotic symptoms that have been already described will make their appearance. Signs of hysteria, anxiety, or some obsession or another may present themselves, which will increase or diminish in relation to the cycle of menstruation, reaching their height a few days before the flow in each month, coincident with it, or when it has ceased. Often the chief manifestation will be a profound depression that may follow a few days of great excitement and euphoria—that is, high spirits, accompanied by a sense of extreme physical fitness.

It is interesting to observe that not only do these signs of emotional disturbance precede the period each month, but they may also appear a year or several months before the courses are established. A fairly regular rhythm may be observed in their appearance and disappearance, while an attack of an hysterical nature, or a few days of great restlessness and irritability, may take place at intervals of about a month. Headaches of the migraine type are also characteristic of the pre-adolescent years, and it is always interesting to keep a note of the date of occurrence of these or any other unusual symptoms that present themselves in girls from ten years old and upwards. In some children menstruation may occur at eleven, while in others it may be delayed until sixteen or seventeen, but the advance or delay is often indicative of precocity, or some retardation of the emotional or intellectual development, which has been slowed down for some reason that is not easy to discover. We may also make some interesting observations between the appearance of menstruation and physical growth, watching when the greatest growth takes place in the individual girl, whether it synchronises with mental development or alternates with it. It is an exceedingly interesting subject, but not much research has been done upon the subject at present.

The alternating exaggerated joy and deep depression that is characteristic of the adolescent is, of course, also typical of many of the manic-depressive states that appear at the other extremity of woman's maturity, that is, the menopause, when they may assume alarming proportions, especially should they have been conspicuous at puberty. For this reason, the girls in whom these manifestations appear should, whenever possible, receive adequate advice and attention. These girls are usually not communicative about their worries or fears. They are naturally shy and reserved, which tendency is increased by the gloom that enwraps them during their period; but the nurse, by showing herself sympathetic, may give them real help at these times, rather than by adopting the vigorous and repellent tone now so often advised by medical women relative to the adolescent girl. This attitude, that the girl who suffers at these times should not be encouraged to make a fuss, because there is nothing to cause any alteration in her life activities in menstruation, is a theory which is typical of many professional women who devote much time and energy to the attempt to deny any differences in physical continuity of health between men and women. They do not wish to acknowledge a difference, because it leaves them with the impression that they come out upon the minus side. This is an excellent example of the dissatisfaction of the woman with her sex, and how it may warp her general opinions throughout her life and work.

For the girl who is disappointed with her life as a woman, this sign of maturity is frequently regarded as a humiliation and a matter of regret. It may, it is true, be connected in her mind with childish wrong-doing, and the threat that it was possible to cause bodily injury if she did not attend to her body as she should, or continued practices that these advisers considered wicked. With the first sign of menstruation, panic often seizes the girl, since to one in whom this feeling of guilt has been implanted it represents proof that the worst has happened, that she is now being punished for her misdeeds, and has probably contracted some terrible disease. Should an adolescent confide fears of this kind to a nurse, she will frequently be able to help her considerably with reassurances, as well as being able to supply her with explanations and information on the subject that may be able to banish the doubts and fears, since the girl will feel that she is obtaining the truth from one who is competent to give her information on this topic.

Notwithstanding the need for adequate elucidation, girls of this age are commonly given very vague explanations about themselves, and what the maturity of life may mean. They tend instead to pick up from one another, their elders or from books, unsavoury notions imparted in any but a wise or favourable way, which causes great havoc in their minds, and prejudices their opinions concerning marriage and childbearing.

The fourth critical stage of the woman's life will come into view at the approach of marriage, which only too often provides a signal for neurotic symptoms to increase, an experience only too familiar to the nurse who has had a number of cases of nerve trouble in her care. It will be interesting for her to notice the particular forms in which neurosis appears, and when listening to the history of the patient's childhood, which will often be confided to her, to draw her own conclusions why the breaking away from home and parents, to make an alliance with a stranger, has led to weakened emotional balance. It may be that the bond to one parent or the other remains too strong for a transference of affection to be made to this new figure, the husband, or that some old childish sense of guilt connected with infantile sexual misdemeanours forms an unconscious barrier against the acceptance of mature sexual life. Similar difficulties in the man's development may also stand in the way of his being an ideal marriage partner, and some definite neurosis, which has hitherto been kept in the background of his life, may now increase so that it cannot be disguised any longer, when adult responsibilities are thrust upon him by marriage.

The nurse requires the utmost tact in dealing with these psycho-neuroses in young married people, and it is essential that she should know something about the probable causes of these critical situations to be able to understand any vague groping for information on the part of her patients, as well as to be able to offer helpful suggestions should her advice be definitely sought. On this point, however, it may be as well here to give the nurse a useful hint upon the matter of giving advice in cases of neurosis. We must remember that in many cases nothing will really help the difficulty but psychological treatment to perform a radical cure, and that advice which merely touches a perplexity in consciousness is comparable with putting vanishing cream upon the surface of the body beneath which is a cancerous growth. Yet, in some less complicated cases of matrimonial mischances, some practical advice on hygiene and matters that may worry those new to marriage may considerably relieve nervous tension. And then, of course, we have always the expedient to hand of giving the really valuable advice to those who wish for it, to seek professional help from the trained expert who will set matters right, and to point out how essential this is for the future health of all concerned, as well as the possible family of the future.

The attitude of many nervously unstable women towards childbearing or breast-feeding their children is one of repulsion, and frequently springs from neurotic fears or childish theories they held long ago concerning the advent of babies, or the mysteries of married life shared by their parents. Strange ideas relative to childbirth survive with curious persistence, although the true facts must have been learned at a later date. For instance, it is by no means uncommon to be told even in these days of enlightenment by mothers that before the birth of their first child they feared they would have to be cut open to effect its birth, believing this to be the normal method of delivery ; and we may conjecture in how many women, who were not very brave, this may have acted as an important deterrent to having, or even to wanting, babies of their own. Motherhood may certainly be regarded for many reasons as one of the most serious danger-zones for the woman, and yet the childless married woman is an extremely frequent sufferer from many forms of neurosis, some of which, in fact, have been known also to contribute their share to hinder childbearing, which has been proved by the occurrence of a quite normal pregnancy and the birth of a healthy child after the cure of the neurosis, which had made the idea of childbearing tolerable.

We have been discussing some of the difficulties that disturb the emotional equilibrium of the married woman, but we must keep before us that psycho-neurosis is equally prevalent or, according to the computation of some medical practitioners, more common among unmarried women. This is far from easy to determine, and the roots of neurosis will be the same in both instances, although in some ways the results and consequences will vary. A few of the determining factors have already been explained; some are too complicated to be suitable for discussion in this simple record, where a deeper knowledge of the underlying mechanisms of neurosis and psycho-neurosis is not presupposed, and so they must be left for further reference should the nurse wish to know more about the subject later on.

In studying the early development of the little girl we drew attention to the fact that she either broke away from her mother as she grew older, in order to transfer the major part of her affection to her father, or she remained fixed by an indestructible bond in childish dependence upon her mother. This alternative constantly furnishes a predisposition to psycho-neurosis, especially when it is made still more complete through the mother's strong attachment to her daughter, accompanied simultaneously by a certain amount of unsatisfied affection existing between the parents, in which case the mother will lavish upon the little girl love that normally should have been divided between husband and child.

Discord between the parents filters into the life of the child through countless small channels that are important, although in themselves they may seem inconspicuous. Through them the child is frequently presented with the perplexing questions, "Whom do I love best, Daddy or Mummy?" "Which of them loves me the most?" Misgivings of this description in the child's mind often sow the seeds of indecision, if not those of serious doubts or obsessions, in which the asking of many questions to gain reassurance will play an important part.

We often find this mother-daughter fixation maintained in successive generations. The mother who was devoted to her own mother may in turn become as deeply attached to her own daughter, bestowing very little affection to her son should she have one. We shall find that each successive stage of separation with the beloved daughter will be attended by a more or less serious breakdown of the mother, and all may be consciously postponed as long as possible. Among these stages of separation we must reckon birth, weaning, the engaging of a nurse, or first going to school; the marriage of the daughter, her wish to take up some profession, or in some cases death. This close tie between mother and daughter, in fact, will often be one of the most significant reasons why the girl does not marry; in the first place because she does not want to leave the mother, and in the second because she is incapable of giving her love to a man. She wants the mother, or a mother substitute alone, which will lead her to form close and emotional friendship with women in whom she will find a reanimation of the mother, or should she also have wished to be a son to the mother instead of a daughter, as is indeed often the case in these complicated instances, she will want to take a man's place in the life of some woman, to love and protect her.

We are familiar with the complexities that arise when the tie between mother and son is too close, but usually the similar state of affairs between mother and daughter is regarded as a charming instance of daughterly devotion, rather than the manifestation of neurosis in both as a rule, that may at any time reach awkward heights for all concerned, and will certainly leave the daughter in a precarious position at the death of the mother.

The mother-daughter fixation in both its aspects will particularly affect the nurse in her professional duties respecting her women patients. When nursing the daughter, she will assuredly be put into the mother's place, and all the old feelings of love will be transferred to her, although an undercurrent of unconscious hatred for the close bondage of the mother may make an appearance in symptomatic actions against the nurse that are by no means understood by the daughter. The situation that arises in the case of nursing the mother, however, is one that offers greater difficulties, especially when the patient is no longer in her first youth. She will then, as inevitably as the daughter, put the nurse into the other position of the dual situation, this time into the place of the daughter, which results in the expectation that she will be able completely to get her to play the part of daughter to the exclusion of independent action, or to be able to fulfil her duties with professional authority.

A further outcome of the transference of affection from daughter to nurse is that the mother may prove rather tyrannical and exacting, and insist that this pseudo-daughter shall obey orders or go. This in itself, as we may easily imagine, will lead to complications, since the nurse usually expects that her patient should follow her lead rather than to issue instructions. But when she holds the clue to the position, by understanding the transference and the power that it has, it will probably be the easier for her to deal with by appearing to carry through the illusion of being the devoted daughter, and skilfully and diplomatically leading when she appears to follow.

We shall be prepared to find this transference to be a positive one (that of love). In the case of an old lady suffering from paranoia or melancholy, however, the nurse might find herself confronted by a negative transference (that of hate, or, as in the paranoic, love transformed by disappointment into hate), so that a lifetime's accumulation of hostility will find an opportunity for discharge upon the nurse. Only too frequently we find the nursing of the elderly mother being actually carried out by a devoted daughter, who is often obliged to bear the brunt of these negative affects, without the possibility of being able to leave in order to transfer her ministrations to a more tractable patient. Difficulties of this sort make the discharge of nursing duties performed for a neurotic relative exceptionally onerous.

The next critical stage in the woman's life, viewed from the aspect of psychological health, is that of the climacteric, which closes the door of so many possibilities in the life of a woman. Few go through this ordeal without some neurotic difficulties, although the common belief that a very large percentage "go completely off their heads" is by no means true. Some certainly suffer at this time far more than they should, because they have been frightened by cautionary tales about its dangers by unwise or ignorant people.

As in the case of puberty, we often find that some degree of psychogenic disintegration precedes definite physical changes by several years. The mental or emotional disturbance that takes place around the period will be accentuated by irritability, sentimentality, and sometimes a tendency to tears with very little provocation from the affairs of the outside world or other people. The attitude towards young people often undergoes interesting changes, or takes on an exaggerated aspect of friendliness or animosity to young folks of one sex or another. Usually we shall find the woman approaching the menopause becoming exacting and jealous of women younger than herself, especially should they be attractive, but lenient or indulgent to young men who are inclined to show her the smallest attention; or we may find the reverse tendency—strange friendships may spring up between the woman of late middle age and quite young girls, whereby the older woman may renew her youth by her interest in the doings of the next generation.

These are usually the women who have lived their lives, and gained pleasure or satisfaction from them, who can rejoice once more with young girls in their youth and beauty. The unfortunate ones who are nearing old age and realise how much they have missed in life are more inclined to grudge the young the opportunities for happiness that lie before them. In these cases we may frequently observe that in countless little ways, insignificant maybe in themselves, they try to prevent them enjoying many small pleasures, or attempt to curtail their freedom for no very definite reason except to exert their power and give themselves a certain amount of grim satisfaction.

The few years that lead the woman over the bridge of this difficult tract, the hazards of which the nurse knows so well from her experience of psychological patients who are no longer young, will reanimate any old neurotic tendencies that may have appeared in the past. Once more hysterical attacks, melancholia, anxiety, persecution phantasies, and obsessions of all kinds tend to swamp many a woman's hold upon psychological or mental equilibrium, unless she obtain some help to steady her during this uncertain period of chaotic transition. For this reason, psychological treatment has been found by experience to make an admirable outlet for accumulating emotion, and serves to provide reassurance for the fears, which are usually manifold, especially the fear of death, that she will often identify with this termination of an important section of her life, in which she may have experienced her greatest happiness, or on account of which she has suffered the most poignant disappointments.

It is, nevertheless, a most curious phenomenon that the women who bewail their loss most strongly at the climacteric are frequently those who have during the rest of their lives taken pains to deny and avoid anything that they feel to be in any way connected with their sexual life. Now that the opportunities are drifting away from them, they turn and bemoan the loss in a way that they themselves seldom recognise as being extremely illogical. That aspect of life for which in the past they have had no use, and which is now drawing to its close, they become sentimental over, calling to mind the old saying, "Blessings brighten as they take their flight." The psychological undercurrent in this case is exceptionally interesting, and may well leave us wondering whether once again we are not face to face with a problem where the mind is thinking two thoughts at once, or saying one thing while it believes another, thus providing us with clear evidence of the functioning of Conscious and Unconscious Minds at one and the same time, the one denying what the other would affirm.

BOOKS THAT MAY BE READ IN CONNECTION WITH THIS CHAPTER

1923. *Mother and Son,* by Gasquoine Hartley.
1925. *Psychoanalyse der Weiblichen Sexualfunctionen,* by Dr. Helene Deutsch.
1930. *Don't be tired,* by Dr. Peter Schmidt

CHAPTER VI

PSYCHOLOGICAL DISORDERS COMMON AMONG MEN AND BOYS

It is popularly supposed that psycho-neuroses are not so frequent among men as among women, but it is doubtful whether accurate statistics would yield corroboration of this belief. Should we make a survey of attendance records of clinics for the treatment of these disorders, the common experience is to find that the numbers of cases of each sex are about equal, although the form of the trouble from which they suffer may be slightly different, whether the patient be a child, an adolescent, or an adult of either sex. Among those whose physical ailments may have been partly determined by neurosis or have been precipitated by some emotional crisis, for which illness provides a temporary escape, we should probably find the numbers equal once again.

The usual supposition is also that hysteria is more prevalent among women and neurasthenia among men, but from the time of John Elliotson onwards (1791–1868) specialists have pointed out that men as well as women suffer from symptoms that are typical of hysteria, and it is by no means uncommon to find neurasthenia figuring upon a medical certificate given to a woman recommending rest from work or to admit her to a convalescent home.

Childhood will provide the same predisposing causes for neurotic disorder in the boy as well as the girl, but we shall find that the boy, who has been made the special pet of his mother and the idol of the home in his early years, may have a more difficult struggle to become adjusted to reality that does not maintain the same flattering attitude towards him than the girl. Usually the boy receives far more adulation of an emotional kind from a larger number of women than the little girl does from the men in her environment, and consequently continues to demand that this shall remain his right throughout life. We find him, as a rule, not so heavily burdened with the necessity of pleasing as the girl, and he seems to have very little of the overwhelming feeling of guilt about his sex that we often find in the girl from an exceedingly early age, especially when disappointment was felt in the family at her birth, because she was not the son who had been so ardently longed for.

The typical attitude of the boy is to be thoroughly satisfied with his sex, and he seldom shows any anxiety to change places with his sister, a desire which we discover commonly enough in many instances at some time or another in the childhood of the little girl. The boy who does wish to be a girl generally has a number of quite definite reasons for wanting to do so, which will be described in detail later on in the chapter.

It is no uncommon experience to learn that the mother from birth onwards derives greater pleasure from services rendered to her son than to her daughter, and shows him more demonstrative affection, which leaves its own mark in the character-formation of the boy as well as that of the girl, who is usually quite capable of noting the differences in their respective treatment even while still in the nursery. The father, on the other hand, will, in a large number of cases, tend to be more jealous of the mother's attentions to the son than to the girl, as well as being inclined to treat him with greater severity for this same reason of unconscious rivalry, unless he should identify himself with this child and feel that what is done for his son is equal to a favour or service rendered to himself. Naturally enough, when we find parents who are not quite normal—that is, free from neurotic trouble—themselves, we may constantly remark that the mother often prefers her daughters and actively dislikes her sons, while the father's preference is similarly contrary to custom because he makes a favourite of his son and ignores his daughters. This reversed situation will commonly shift all the emotional accents of the family balance. It will also disturb the normal course of growing-up by identification with the parent of the same sex, while the major portion of the child's love is expended upon the parent of the opposite sex, which paves the way for the characteristic preferences of adult life, when the time comes for choosing a marriage partner.

The deeply mother-fixated little boy usually shows a strong disinclination to grow up, because he sees quite clearly that this will mean separation from his mother by gradual stages. The mother, who is also as devoted to the little son, may be as reluctant for the time to come when he ceases to be the *mother's baby*, and frequently without being aware of the serious consequences that may follow her actions, or the dangerous influence they may exert upon the future, puts numberless stumbling-blocks in his way.

Peter Pan as a nursery hero has unfortunately shown many little boys that others besides themselves have the same wish, which in the story certainly seems to be one that is entirely laudable, that of not wanting to grow-up, but to stay eternally a child. In this picturesque child-hero they see the little god, and many will swiftly incorporate this new version among their own phantasies which have arisen since infancy, the focus of which has remained unchanged, to be the deity enthroned upon his mother's lap. This being the case, we may readily see how the favourite pictures of a modern Christ-child and Madonna, with which we so freely decorate our nurseries, help to establish the same idea yet more firmly, and to construct what psycho-analysts call the God Complex in the minds of our little boys, which is the outcome of primary Self-love or narcissism.

Not only do we discover in these children the wish not to grow-up, not to learn how to do things for themselves, which would naturally destroy the need of having eager, helpful worshippers, but we notice concurrently an insatiable thirst for admiration, outspoken praise, and compliments. It is also usual to find that these children in whom the God Complex is inordinately strong are of the type specially admired in this country, the fair, curly-haired, angel-faced little boys we so often find used as models in the modern versions of the Christ-child that have recently made their appearance in such large numbers. These children from their earliest days have thus been recipients of much adulation and many compliments, which create in them the need for this gratification to such an extent that they suffer from a sense of deprivation should the supply not always be sustained at a constant level.

This curtailment of admiration may be caused in several ways. Firstly, the parents may suddenly become aware that the child is expecting it and decide that it must stop, without reflecting that such a sudden and drastic cessation of narcissistic gratification is likely to have an injurious result. Frequently it will force the child to seek some new or exaggerated way of showing off in order to continue to gain the praise that formerly came freely and unasked. Sometimes it will be gained through illness, or the child's reaction will be to withdraw into itself and become intensely unhappy over this abrupt withdrawal of what has been considered the usual manifestation of love from those around him. Therefore to the child mind the absence of admiration signifies the loss of love. Another frequent cause of this change in attitude with its diminution of attention is the arrival of a little brother or sister who deflects the admiration, so that the interest of the household or of passers-by will be concentrated entirely on the new-comer, or at any rate will have to be shared.

Such disappointments in the life of the little boy often form the beginnings of neurotic trouble and show themselves later in different ways according to the temperament of the child. Other factors will also contribute their share, chief among which, perhaps, may be reckoned the age of the child, the sex of the supplanter, and the amount of adulation that was received in the past in relation to the extent of the deprivation in the present.

As we have already pointed out, unhappiness quickly undermines the child's resistance to both physical disease and infection. During illness the lost attention will naturally be recovered, and the child who is seriously ill will immediately become the centre of interest to the exclusion of all rivals. In this way we may see that even in childhood the secondary gain of illness is in operation. The little boy of the "beautiful type," which has already been mentioned, is sure to attract admiration and demonstrations of affection from nurses who look after him at home or in hospital, as well as from other patients, should he unfortunately find himself in an adult ward rather than one for children only, which accident merely adds one more stage to the neurotic opportunities of his life.

Schooldays will bring further troubles in their wake. Going to school necessitates the separation from mother and home, should this not have been accomplished even partially by any other means before, and the introduction to schoolfellows, some of whom will be older than himself and many of whom may actively envy and dislike him for his appearance that is so unlike their own. His manner of expecting admiration and deference, together with the general air of superiority which he adopts in regard to other children, will usually make for unpopularity and lead to experiences that will be by no means pleasant. Following this first break from home we frequently find the signal for the appearance of some form of child neurosis, or its conversion into diffused ill-health of some kind, which will necessitate leaving school for the time being, with its many unwelcome factors, and the return home to resume the old conditions of love, understanding, and power.

Another unconscious method used by these children for escaping from an outside world that does not come up to expectations, and a reality which leaves so much to be desired, is the little boy's substitution of phantasy for reality in his day-dreams, or the wonderful stories about his own doings which he will recount to others, which tendency is known as *pseudologia phantastica*. Gradually, in face of the increasing difficulties of real achievement, the need for these phantasies of imaginary great doings becomes more urgent, until we may find in extreme cases the child living almost entirely in a phantasy world of his own, retreating from reality with its unwished-for requirements. This forms the central growing-point in severe cases, whence Dementia Præcox may develop in a recognisable form at adolescence or in the early twenties, when reality shows the boy a still more drastic necessity to confront life's problems. The final refusal on his part, when retreat into a complete phantasy life takes place, is a most grave condition from which in most cases there will be no return, although very early cases in childhood may be successfully treated by psychological methods.

It is customary to find among phantasies of the Dementia Præcox type those with which we have become familiar in connection with the God Complex that has been mentioned before, those of greatness, importance, being possessed of magical power or of supernatural influence over the elements. There is, however, another characteristic group that represents an escape from the real home to find another more compatible with the desire to be the one and only loved person, actually the baby in the cradle, or even before birth. In these a nest, an island, or a little hole in the ground will be imagined, where the child lives all alone or is perhaps looked after by one person or creature, whom we may easily recognise as the mother or a mother in disguise of a bird, a tender-hearted animal, as well as Wendy in the Peter Pan legend.

The withdrawal from the real world into the self, which is found typified in these phantasies, will often have yet another manifestation, that of autœrotic gratification, sometimes taking place in conjunction with the phantasies, at others occurring whenever the little boy feels particularly unhappy, lonely, or inefficient. This tendency to masturbation, which is so often referred to under the name of bad habits, will more commonly be found occupying a prominent place among the early neurotic symptoms of a little boy than of his sister, for several reasons, although it is true that it is frequently passed unnoticed in the girl.

Chief among these will be the fact that it is more generally detected in the boy, and that comparatively severe measures are taken to check it. These will often be combined with exceedingly unwise threats of punishment that arouse guilt and fear, although they will frequently not have the desired effect of eradication, but serve to stamp it more indelibly on the child's mind, and leave a burden of anxiety which is always liable to come to the surface throughout life connected with any sort of situation that may cause the child to feel guilty.

Threats and punishment relative to masturbation are usually associated with the boy's father, and with the child's love to the mother, who often gives the child the first stimulation of the kind in her earliest ministration of washing and toilet operations, so that it is by no means uncommon to notice that the guilt and fear involved in masturbation will be inextricably connected with the child's attitude to both parents and ideas of love, hatred, and rivalry that exist as an undercurrent of the family triangle.

As we should rightly suppose, the symptoms connected with this habit of masturbation, that arise partly from threats that have been used to check it, will be highly charged with guilt and fear concerning this symbol of masculinity, namely, the penis, for which the little fellow gets into such dire disgrace for touching or playing with, in what is presented to him as an illicit manner. A frequent fear that arises from this is that his organ may be hurt, or even forfeited, for the continued wrong-doing, which gives rise to many other allied fears and anxiety symptoms in the boy's life.

The fear of the father and the guilt attached to the boy himself may often turn into hatred and create repressed wishes for revolt against the father, which later on will be transferred to those who occupy a corresponding position in respect to him, being in a position of authority, and able to reprimand or punish him for wrong-doing. In some cases this fear causes the child to wish himself a girl, so that he would then not only be without this particular source of temptation, giving way to which both angers the father and draws down punishment upon himself, but also because the boy feels that as a little daughter he might attract the love of the father instead of his severity. When this idea occurs to the mind of the child we will often find him adopting a more or less feminine attitude towards the two parents, turning away from the mother, whom he may now regard with jealousy as a rival where the love of his father is concerned, and seeking the affection of the father with the most obvious anxiety, while he makes deliberate efforts to please him.

This naturally is not the sign that we welcome for the future healthy development of the boy. It is frequently attended by trouble at school and elsewhere, because the boy will continue to seek over-emotional friendships with men and boys older than himself who take the father's place, and in later life he shuns the more normal society of girls of his own age, amongst whom normally he might have found a future mate. The tendency of the boy to love members of his own sex only will generally spring from one of three main sources, thus:

(*a*) The boy loves other boys because originally he loved himself only. Thus in his affection for other boys he is still, through identification, loving himself, like Narcissus, who fell in love with his own image reflected in the water. For this reason it is called *narcissistic homosexuality.*

(*b*) The boy wants the affection of other men or boys older than himself, who will behave towards him as he formerly wished his father to treat him, i.e. as the favourite little daughter. (Passive homosexuality.)

(*c*) The boy wants to play the father or mother to a boy younger than himself, who is going to be a picture of himself as he once was, when some person whose love he valued bestowed it upon him unstintingly. (Active homosexuality.) This tendency will usually be found constructed as follows, (Sigmund Freud. Collected Papers, Vol. II. *Certain Neurotic Mechanisms in Jealousy, Paranoia, and Homosexuality.*)

The little boy was in the first place deeply attached to his mother, but was alienated from her at some time for one of various reasons. He was disappointed with her to find that she was a woman, therefore she had no penis, which he himself values so highly, and as such is an inferior being. A second cause of trouble where the mother is concerned may arise because he feels that she has deserted him by having another baby, whom apparently she loves more than himself, or because she has preferred and praised a rival. The idea of rivalry is always painful to the little boy, whether this rival is younger than oneself, i.e. the baby, a contemporary or someone older, the father or an elder brother. There is also another cause which sometimes accounts for the little boy's turning away from the mother at the birth of the brother or sister. This usually will only be felt vaguely and for an exceedingly brief period. Then it is swiftly and deeply repressed. The cause of the trouble will be that he is jealous that the mother and not he has produced this wonderful baby, and, moreover, he learns that he in person will never be able to bear a child.

In order to escape from the pain of rivalry caused by hearing the mother's praise bestowed upon another, the little boy may cease to love her, with or without hating her, as the case may be. He thereupon makes alliance with the rival in order to save himself the pangs of jealousy, and in turn seeks another boy rather younger than himself, whom he may love as he felt his mother formerly loved him. The other alternative is to split himself into two and thus become a representative of the loving mother as well as the loved child, so that in future he loves himself only and takes a maternal care of himself, his health, or general welfare. He may also try to escape from the gnawing jealousy caused by realising that his mother can do more wonderful things than he, in that she has borne a child, by finding some little boy or girl to "mother," who becomes his phantasy child. This occasionally may be the little supplanter, but it is more usual for another child in no way connected with the family to take this rôle, for obvious reasons.

This wish to bear the child, as origin or motive of the *mother tendency*, will practically always remain unconscious, but it will have several interesting consequences. It may lead to a highly developed urge to give expression to the creative instinct, and we find the child always trying to make something, not anxious to part with anything that has been made, but to gain praise for the activity. He will want to find out about the origins of things and how they are made, show a tendency to destroy what others have constructed or to belittle them, showing that unconscious jealousy is still active in results. The disappointment in childhood will also find gratification in actual perversion, or in a sublimated form through befriending little boys, working with Scouts, or Boy's Clubs, and such-like. In its crude form, of course, we shall find it taking the unwished-for route of illicit behaviour with boys younger than himself, on account of which he may get himself as well as his little companions into serious trouble at school.

These abnormal trends in development which we see during childhood in a larval state will account for a high percentage of the psycho-neuroses that we find in boys at adolescence or in adult life. We may now retrace our steps briefly to discover how they will affect mature development and what they will provide in the form of neurotic symptoms or behaviour that would cause difficulties during illness or convalescence for the nurse. At this point it may also be as well to remind readers that in this chapter many of the difficulties and origins of nervous troubles in the boy have been omitted, which have already been mentioned in former chapters, for the sake of excluding unnecessary repetition as much as possible. When symptoms arising from the same cause and having a similar origin are found in males as well as females it seems needless to give their details more than once. But it is well to keep in mind that boys who have distinct inclinations to girlishness and women with a masculine tendency will frequently follow a course of development which we may have described in the psycho-neuroses which are more common in the other sex. It should also be understood that unfortunately it is quite impossible to describe and explain the origin of all the neurotic symptoms and manifestations that can be found among our patients;

many must necessarily be excluded on account of available space.

The little boy's fixation to his mother, the conflict between wanting to grow up and the desire to remain a baby, in order to keep her to himself and to banish the father, who, although he may not show manifest jealousy, certainly exercises some discipline over the little fellow, leads to the same hysterical symptoms that we described appearing in the little girl, in many cases. We will also find general and specific fears, anxiety, hysteria, doubts, and obsessions, plus those which typically arise in the boy who has learned guilt and fear through threats connected with masturbation. The attempt to gain more love from the mother, to keep her love or to bring it back should it show signs of becoming diverted to another, for instance, a new baby, may cause some form of physical illness in childhood that will tend to repeat at any subsequent time, when events show signs of re-animating similar dangers to those which caused the step to be taken during the early childhood. These often go through a second stage at adolescence, if not before. Adolescence has already been shown to be a period of psychological repetition, when all childish neurotic symptoms are liable to be reanimated, and a still later series may be apparent after marriage, when the wife will often consciously or unconsciously take the mother's place to her husband.

In this connection we should bear in mind that the boy who originally was and who remained too deeply attached to his mother, especially when the fixation is held equally fast from her side also, may in many cases be unable to find any woman as wife who could fulfil all his requirements. He frequently, in point of fact, does not marry at all, but continues to live with his mother, after his father's death, when the original child-wish naturally will gain real satisfaction; or should he marry he will most probably never be content unconsciously, even if consciously he is not aware of the wish that his wife does not treat him as the baby he still really desires to be. Should this be the case, it will follow that he is usually unwilling to have children of his own, because eventually they would usurp his place. He would be jealous of them should they arrive, and might frequently become ill when they were born, partly in identification with their mother, or, again, if they seemed likely to divert too much of her time and thoughts away from himself.

How may this tendency to repeat the original situation in illness, being regression to childhood as well as a determined attempt to snatch the first place, affect the patient's behaviour during illness? We may trace the plan of old events fairly completely through our own observation of the male patients we have nursed. It is habitual to find that the average nurse says she prefers nursing men to women, giving as her reason that they are *easier* to nurse. This may well be so, because as a rule the man quickly transfers to her all the old feelings of love and confidence that he once entertained for his mother as a child, and revives the belief that if she looks after him he will soon be restored to health.

In the nurse he will once more find the loving mother, or sometimes the severe one, and he often transfers his suspicion and dislike originally felt in connection with his father to the doctor. It is more than likely that he will be jealous of any other patients whom the nurse is attending at the same time, and try to be preferred for some reason, or more ill and therefore more necessitous of her care than they. If he is being nursed alone at home, or privately in a nursing-home, the jealousy will of necessity be directed upon past or future patients. The chief drawback to the successful nursing of these cases will be the Peter Pan tendencies of childhood, which will show a serious recrudescence, so hindering recovery or convalescence, during which growing-up has symbolically to be carried out for a second time before adult life can be resumed, and when finally the nurse, the substitute mother, again disappears and her devoted attendance upon him ceases.

It is this type of man who will frequently wish to marry his nurse in order that he may keep her always beside him, so that he need never completely grow up. Then, whatever may befall him in life, he will always have her at hand to help him. This dependence upon the nurse probably reaches its maximum in the condition of anxiety neurosis, where doubts that need reassurance are essential factors. Yet we find in many cases that the patients who suffer from obsessional neurosis often show a tendency to identification with the opposite sex. That being so, the patient being a man, his feminine inclination would sometimes cause him to seek sympathy and reassurance from the male doctor rather than from the nurse. But the more usual experience is that an ambivalent attitude obtains to doctor and nurse; first one will be wanted and then another, or perhaps both, and we shall discover the conditions of the patient's preference, or the causes of turning from the one to the other. The man with an obsessional neurosis will repeatedly show his unconscious negative feelings to the medical man, by inability to be comforted or convinced by his advice. He will continue to wonder whether he has not made a mistake or overlooked an important symptom in the illness which would materially alter the diagnosis. Doubts of this description repeatedly send these patients from one end of Harley Street to the other, or upon fruitless visits to all the hospitals in London, their fears only pacified for the time being, and then once more they become assailed with doubt, which urges them to set out afresh to find someone new whom they feel confident understands their case.

An interesting reanimation of a certain type of childish behaviour will once more be seen in the married man with regard to his nurse during illness, which it may be well to explain in detail, since it is one that very often leads to misunderstandings all round. We have already explained that the married man may become ill when his wife has given him some occasion for jealousy where she herself or her children are concerned. The jealous person frequently tries to pay others back in the same coin; therefore nothing is easier than to try to accomplish this by using the nurse as a convenient weapon. The husband, feeling sore at his wife's neglect, although consciously he may not realise that this is the source of his trouble, hails the advent of the nurse with pleasure. He feels that here at last is another woman whose mission in life for the present, at all events, is simply and solely to attend to his wants and wishes. The consequence may be that he will take especial pains to show his wife how much more attentive, skilled, and interesting the nurse is in every way than herself, particularly if she should have been trying to nurse him for a few days with very little time and not much skill before it was decided to call in a professional nurse. The nurse also in the depths of her unconscious mind may not be at all averse to show herself infinitely superior to another woman, and eagerly takes part in the game prepared by her patient, with the result that a small or great drama is no unlikely occurrence, which usually causes considerable unhappiness to all concerned before it is played out and matters are set right again.

The guilt and results of threats consequent upon childish or adolescent masturbation will reverberate in the exhaustion of neurasthenia as well as in the depression associated with melancholia, in which guilt, apparently attached to some entirely vague and abstract wrong-doing, generally forms the nucleus of the illness. It is curious to note how closely the symptoms usually complained of by those suffering from neurasthenia follow the model of sensations observed by the boy in himself after he has been masturbating, especially if he had read of its supposed ill effects, or has been threatened with its "terrible consequences" by someone who has been trying to frighten him out of the habit. In point of fact we will usually find that this early nervous symptom has played an important part in the life of practically all persons, male or female, who later on develop true neurasthenia, although the term is often loosely applied to forms of hysteria, being considered a less invidious term, by those who are not exceedingly accurate in their scientific nomenclature. This fact, however, will generally be kept from the knowledge of the nurse, who consequently is left to draw her own conclusions from what she may hear indirectly or from her knowledge of the history of other cases.

It would nevertheless be a considerable help to her in her professional duties should they include the nursing of men and boys, especially during adolescence, to equip herself with some of the little pamphlets designed to teach the boy "purity," or to check "self-abuse," as well as to give them information of what a young boy ought to know. She may read these carefully as well as one or two others of a more reliable nature, the titles of which will be given in the list at the end of this chapter, so that she may compare fiction with fact, to see how the combination of guilt and fear has caused the suggestions contained in the books to take effect until some of these symptoms are actually believed to be present. They will become established owing to the old substructure of guilt more easily than they can afterwards be removed. Sometimes this may be accomplished by giving the boy accurate information concerning matters that have perplexed him, but in the majority of cases it will be necessary to make use of thorough psychological treatment before the harm that has already been done can be eradicated.

Matrons or nurses in Preparatory and Public Schools are usually not particularly well equipped in this respect concerning knowledge of the troubles and conflicts that are going on in the minds and bodies of their young patients. For this reason they are unable to deal with them adequately should need arise to give advice or information at this difficult age, especially since those seeking it show their requirements but vaguely and fumblingly. We should also remember that it will not only be lack of knowledge of this subject which causes many nurses trouble in exposition of this subject, but also the two factors of their own sexual repressions and maybe their unresolved complexes concerning envy of the opposite sex.

In the group of neurotic disturbances that we have already described in connection with symptoms which at their worst develop into dementia præcox, we shall find all stages of phantasy development, pathological lying (pseudologia phantastica), and juggling with reality, which form a bridge by way of pathological doubt, with obsessional neurosis, in which hallucinations may be seen, heard, or felt. When this group of disorders reach a highly developed stage, so that they frequently are reckoned among the psychoses—that is, the insanities, or as incipient insanity—they come more within the province of the nurse with medico-psychological training rather than one who has a general certificate; and yet, since it is by no means uncommon to meet with some of these symptoms or their traces accompanying physical disorders, and acting as their serious complications, it may be well to give some brief descriptions of the most frequent forms in which they will occur. Among this perplexing group we may also allocate those patients who are afflicted with psycho-genic epilepsy (see p 145), since their symptoms as well as motives are similar in many respects, such as the desire to escape from the troublesome world and the people in it who are felt to be so conspicuously wanting in understanding.

Thus it is a usual experience that patients with a tendency

to introversion, that is, who are absorbed in themselves to the exclusion of the outer world and the people in it, such as occurs in dementia præcox and severe melancholia, will require much sleep and wake with difficulty in the morning, because fundamentally they are unwilling to face the new day and the fresh events it may bring. Their convalescence will be equally slow, and they will incline to hug the disease which makes such an effectual barrier between them and the realities of life. In later stages of these psychoses we shall find conditions of coma, catatonia, and hebephrenia, where very little contact with the outer world remains, and although still alive the patient shows no interest in the affairs taking place around him, nor does he make any sign that he notices people, unless these should disturb him in any way, which may provoke sudden and violent anger for a time. Phantasy will in minor cases gradually replace reality until delusions of grandeur or magic will absorb the greater part of the conscious thoughts, so that realisation that these phantasies bear little or no relation to truth is scanty.

We may sometimes find that these patients have always been inactive since babyhood, always ready to sink back into slumber, from which they were aroused with extreme difficulty. In some cases we hear that they were infants in whom, after birth, it was extremely difficult to establish respiration. The lifelong tendency to inertia draws them back to the nest, the little island, or the hole in the ground of their phantasies, which symbolises for them the uterus in which they were content for so long, alive although no exertion was required of them.

The unhappiness of the little boy who felt unwanted or neglected by his environment will be found once more in the melancholic patient. This form of psycho-neurosis is prevalent among men in late middle age, although it may often be camouflaged skilfully as anxiety about business, the welfare of their families, or what would happen to their wives if they were to die unexpectedly. The fear that others would be hard put to it to manage without them is the direct outcome of an old wish to be wanted by someone, and the sad feeling that they mattered to nobody. They may have the one complaint for ever on their lips that they are of no use in the world any more, or that nothing seems worth while now. These thoughts are typical of the man who has retired from business or his profession, and who therefore has little to do which really interests him, after leading a busy, interesting life. Through his worries he provides considerable distress for his friends and relations; many will drift away from him, alienated by his constant complaints or his continual grumbles that others treat him badly, whilst those who cannot get away find life in his environment exceedingly depressing.

These melancholic patients often find a last solution of their troubles in suicide or fatal accident, which is a similar means of gaining an escape from their own maladjustment to life. Again, observation shows us that a certain amount of religious mania will often be connected with this acute depression, but it will run concurrently with the other symptoms of the disease and does not tend to benefit the patient's condition. It seldom provides any satisfactory solution of difficulties, however, since the wish for power that frequently, when ungratified, forms the basis of melancholy and the exaggerated guilt that accompanies it represents a cardinal hindrance to accepting a religious power that is greater than the patient's own, or an authority that can grant absolution to so great a sinner. This self-importance attached to guilt thus makes a barrier which prevents any satisfactory cure, since it is usually easier to attract attention and interest through being ill than by being in normal health.

Another serious obstacle that occurs in these patients

as well as those suffering from dementia præcox is that they have already withdrawn their capacity to be interested too far from reality to be influenced by another person, so that the transference, which is essential for psychological methods of cure, which take place largely through identification, cannot eventuate, unless the treatment is commenced early, before this regression has advanced so far. When the patient is completely readjusted to this limited existence, with all his interest concentrated on his illness, his misery, and misfortune, it is impossible to enable him to see that in many cases the present condition is a wish-fulfilment and has little reality outside his own making, and represents a method of atonement for some unconscious guilt, or is a repetition of an early trauma of disappointment.

We cannot hope to alleviate this grave condition of neurotic illness unless some small remnant of transference capacity remains, which will attach itself to the nurse as a manifestation of the father-daughter situation, representing an original mother-son fixation. The standard disappointment originally felt over the withdrawal of love on the part of the mother might then be knit together once again, but we should probably find that the patient would want to keep this nurse, upon whom he had come to rely, permanently. In practice we will often find an elderly man who develops some morbid condition which requires the constant attention of the nurse, which gives him the possibility to fulfil his wish. The complete cure of persons considerably past middle age who suffer from acute neuroses or psycho-neuroses may scarcely be hoped for, except in very rare cases. But we frequently observe that understanding treatment or nursing founded upon psychological knowledge carried out by a nurse who is conversant with the principles underlying the construction of neurotic diseases will greatly relieve nervous tension and provide outlets for the accumulation of emotions arising from the mechanisms supplying the symptoms, which is, after all, more than will be accomplished in other ways as a rule.

When we were discussing the little boy's attitude towards the father, and attempting to show that it might at times produce a twofold tendency of love and hate, sometimes closely interwoven, at others alternating, we remarked that this conflict between love and hate frequently gives rise to other forms of neurosis besides the direct tendency to a homosexual attraction that we have already described at some length. In the first instance, we may mention the obsessional neuroses, in which we find the magic rituals being carried out to prevent misfortune expected from another (the father usually), or to counteract injury that may have been inadvertently or otherwise caused by oneself to another (the father or mother). These symptoms usually disguise death-wishes that have been the outcome of hatred and fear of someone who is stronger than the child, and from whom revenge is expected for wrong-doing, that may not have been carried farther than thought, but on account of which very great guilt is experienced nevertheless.

The consequent guilt, fear, and hatred will often account for the other manifestations that we associate with obsessional neuroses, the ambivalence (mixed attitude of hatred and love), the doubt, the wish for reassurances of all kinds, the magical words or actions used to prevent danger to others, or to preserve the self from others. These compulsive actions or thoughts may often cause tics, which will in themselves be a vehicle for several repressed ideas, thus they may form an equivalent of organ-speech, and express through gesture an idea that could not be spoken in words, or they may provide a form of auto-erotic pleasure through alternation of muscular tension and relaxation. The latter will occasionally take the place of, and furnish a substitute for, genital masturbation in a disguised form that may be practised openly for this reason in defiance of parental prohibitions. Some forms of stammer may be of a similar nature, with the addition of oral components, which thus find expression in alliance with demonstrations of fear, hatred, and guilt once experienced in relation to the angry father.

As one may imagine, the nurse does not play such an important part in these forms of male neurosis as in those where the mother was the central figure. But in consequence of the ætiology of the neurosis—the rivalry of the father where the mother was concerned, which caused anxiety in connection with the father, so that love felt towards the mother was deflected from the normal situation in order to escape possible retaliation—the nurse may eventually show the way back to a normal state of health. During the cure she may find herself playing a progressively important part where her male patients are concerned, as the disorder is being traced back through the abnormal layers of love for the father in order to reach earlier and more normal phases of mother love that must be released from inhibition before it can once more be liberated and bestowed upon a wife in a mature way. For this reason it is essential that patients who require nursing while they are undergoing psychological treatment shall have about them nurses who are in favour of it and understand its process. Furthermore, it is still more beneficial if they have sufficient knowledge concerning the course of psychological treatment to be able to follow the reactions of the patients when one stage succeeds another. This needs a realisation of the way in which the treatment revives one phase after another of childhood development, that will be accompanied by the corresponding emotions respecting those about them, whom they place as substitutes for father, mother, brothers, and sisters.

Among the group of neuroses prevalent among men that are mainly derivatives of the child's original attitude to the father, we must certainly not omit paranoia, alcoholism, and drug addiction. It has been suggested when an explanation of paranoia in women was given that it usually arises in connection with persons of the same sex, and that the former dearly loved parent or a substitute finally becomes, through disappointment, the persecuting agent, and the source whence danger is expected. We shall find this same mechanism present in the homosexual tendency, which characteristically shows itself in a great esteem or admiration for someone in an important position, an employer, a minister of religion, a social worker, perhaps a medical man. For a time this person is regarded with the utmost reverence and devotion, but then, when this parent substitute causes disappointment, once more through failure of response, the former positive attitude changes to one of hatred, which includes fear of what the person is going to do. Suspicions of persecution, of planned injury, phantasies of ill-treatment, are rapidly organised, and the patient may complain to friends in veiled terms at first, which frequently become more clear as the disorder increases in severity, of the unkindness of this person or of a mysterious persecution carried on by persons unknown. He may then proceed to write anonymous letters to the supposed persecutor or denounce him formally to the police, imploring their protection or demanding that steps shall be taken to bring the miscreant to justice. Ideas of spies, secret societies, or magic influences are frequent in these phantastic delusions, from which the patient himself suffers untold misery, and before long many of those who try to help him in his troubles will be involved in the confusion. The patient's wife is frequently drawn in to play a leading part in this drama of delusion. She will be regarded as unfaithful, the accomplice of the same person to whom the patient himself is emotionally attracted, the former friend. No proofs to the contrary, nor protests on the part of the suspected persons, avail to clear up the suspicions, and the end of the trouble will usually be the removal of the patient to some mental home or institution suitable for the care of such people so that others besides themselves may be protected from the dangerous results of their delusions.

The subject of alcoholism and drug addiction has received considerable attention of late years in connection with the renewed interest that the discovery of psycho-analysis has focused upon all abnormal mental or nervous conditions. On the one hand it has been shown to be a regression to the early oral stages, when the mouth of the infant supplied all that was necessary for contentment, and the mother herself was impersonal as long as she continued to supply the necessary adjunct of happiness. When this source failed, and the mother through refusal became an opposing, and therefore a more personal object, hatred followed. The mother was hated, and the love that might once have been unconsciously associated with the food received, and then transferred to the person who supplied it, was withdrawn first into the self and then given to others like the self. Later on fresh means of securing oral gratification were found in alcohol, that served not only to show complete independence of the mother, but proved also a cause of annoyance to her. This enabled the child, now grown-up, to feel his freedom from the restraint of the mother, as well as through the action of the alcohol to liberate himself to break down inhibitions so as to become abusive or violent towards the mother herself, women in general, or a particular mother substitute, fiancée or wife.

Very frequently we find that men who are addicted to alcohol make a conscious excuse that they want to banish disappointment or worry, which actually is a revival of the original situation. Another characteristic of alcoholism is that usually it will be partaken of in the company of other male contemporaries at some social gathering, that often excludes the society of women, and that men who are intoxicated usually indulge in stories unflattering to women or become abusive of them, while they magnify their own abilities or the general superiority of their own sex. This frequency with which intoxicated men fabricate wonderful doings, resembling the manifestations of pseudologia phantastica, and those that are unflattering or degrading to women, suggests by the exaggerated effect shown that this is a reaction-formation to cover the sense of inferiority they felt in their childhood relative to the mother. Their favourite theme of the frailty of women's morals suggests also the power they wish to feel they can exercise over them, and leads us to conclude that the effect of alcohol raises barriers of repression which allows them to show their primitive wishes represented by their stories. We may also see reflected their infantile attitude of needing to join with others before they can voice their disapproval of woman to degrade her in revenge for the old disappointments and her training which attempted to teach them self-control. If she is as depraved as they wish to make it appear, where, then, is the superiority she tried to show in the past? She is really no better than they, after all!

It is interesting to note that the woman's attitude towards the man who is addicted to alcohol is usually a corresponding reaction to his unconscious motive, since we shall find her disgusted and repulsed by it, as though she knew that it was an act of revenge against herself.

The woman alcoholic, however, has generally a strong identification with men, and wishes to imitate them in their own oral gratification. She likes to drink with them on equal terms of companionship, but at the same time will often show herself deeply attracted by members of her own sex, to whom she wishes to play the man's part. She seeks to dominate them and obviously finds through the influence of the intoxicant a raising of her repressions, similar to that of the man under the same conditions, which enables her to gratify her wishes to a greater extent than she would otherwise feel at liberty to do.

It is instructive to watch the mechanisms at work in the woman who seeks to cure a man of alcoholic addiction and observe the ways in which she tries to substitute herself for the craving for liquor or drugs. Unconsciously she has the right idea in her head, but she does not know precisely how to combat the very great difficulties that lie before her, because of the construction of the addiction. The principal factor of the obstacle that lies before her in this struggle is that it represents the man's infantile hostility to the woman, his desire to offend, degrade, and disgust her. Naturally it serves to reawaken all these old feelings with redoubled force directly she shows her wish to establish her control over him through a second deprivation of this precious fluid, which he now feels furnishes him with all that life can offer him by way of compensation for its trials and disappointments, as in the past the mother denied him her breast.

The drugs that are taken by mouth will show approximately the same mechanisms, but frequently point to a deeper repression or an earlier stage than when the substitute gratification takes the form of alcohol taken in the company of others. The action is more analogous to the urge of the secret drinker, being without the definite homosexual component provided by the convivial companions, or the gross manifestations of hostility shown as the accompaniments of the use of intoxicating liquors. Drugs, however, have the same effect of helping their victim to escape temporarily from reality and the unpleasant duties of life into a roseate, dreamy state of infant life without cares, effort, or responsibility; but suggest to us the man contented with himself alone, which is a survival of primary narcissism, rather than the homosexual stage that requires additional stimulation from the presence of others of the same sex for full enjoyment.

Drugs that are administered in other ways than by the mouth take on a certain amount of symbolism from their special method of administration, but the unconscious trends that lie beneath them are too complicated for adequate explanation in this handbook and must be left to the more specialised medical treatise.

The few pages that remain of this chapter are needed to give some brief survey of Traumatic Neurosis, which is to some extent comparable to Occupational Neurosis, that has already been described in the last chapter, and of shell- or war-shock, which brought psycho-neuroses in general into great medical prominence as well as into public notice during and after the Great War. They may here be dealt with together, because conditions that affect the one will usually be found exerting important influence upon the other. At first they were supposed to have this characteristic in common, that their onset was sudden and their cause one isolated shock, so intense that the neurotic condition resulted from that alone. Important factors concerned in the cure, the duration of symptoms, their increase and decrease were observed to be similar when both states of ill-health were scrutinised with close attention.

Thus it was observed that compensation, pension, or damages tended to increase the extent or violence of the symptoms, paralysis, contractures, lameness, inability to talk, blindness, etc., as long as the continuance of payment or amount of payment depended upon the persistence of the injury; that the symptoms themselves were inclined to become more acute during medical examination relative to award of compensation or should a military patient come before an Examining Board relative to extension of treatment allowance or continuance of pension. When these ordeals were safely over, the condition improved until the next became imminent.

It naturally follows that in these cases cure is extremely difficult. During the war a multitude of devices for the treatment of shell-shock were in use: electricity, suggestion, "persuasion," hypnotism. Some of these methods were put into practice immediately the symptoms had appeared as first aid, and sometimes they were successful in that the symptoms were removed for the time being and the patients were sent back to the line. But subsequent experience proved that relapse was frequent in these cases. Once again, corroborating the observation of Bernheim, it was found that those patients with a very simple mentality, who were used to obey orders without criticism or hesitation, were most quickly and easily cured by these expedients, whereas men of a more highly developed intellect, who were less prepared to believe or to do all that they were told without question, were not so readily influenced by such forms of simple therapy. An additional disadvantage to the efficacy of the cure arose from the fact that those who were making use of these methods were themselves only too often still in an experimental stage, without much knowledge of the technique. The same drawback was also apparent with many who then for the time experimented with psycho-analysis, little realising how much there was to be learned about its exceedingly complicated technique. They would often complain of the lack of success of this form of treatment, but apparently did not know enough about it to imagine that the fault might lie with themselves.

Each country involved in the Great War had this same problem to face, and each attempted to do so according to the means and methods at its disposal. Many books were brought out describing treatments or the ætiology of war-shock, which now show an interesting series of advances from the old to the new methods. The first to be published reproduced the methods and technique that had survived for a hundred years or more, such as hypnotism, then the electric current, suggestion with or without hypnotism, and lastly we found some of the younger and more adventurous medical men making use of the methods and discoveries of various comparatively recently introduced forms of psycho-therapy, including psycho-analysis.

Shell-shock in course of time became allocated among the psycho-neuroses, and evidence was advanced to show that only in rare cases could no previous tendency to neurotic trouble be found in the history of the patient, and that it usually represented a recurrence of former trouble, that now appeared as anxiety neurosis, conversion hysteria, or the like, which acted as a defence mechanism against return to the trenches and the horrors of war.

An interesting experiment was carried out on German soldiers suffering from shell-shock by Dr. Ernst Simmel, who revived the cathartic treatment, discovered by Dr. Joseph Breuer (see p. 44), with considerable success. He used to hypnotise several at a time lying on large mattresses covering the floor, and there allow them to abreact their emotions, which the stress of battle or the emotions aroused by war conditions had aroused without providing adequate discharge.

In England many forms of Occupation Therapy were attempted. In some localities special institutions for the purpose were established, but they do not seem to have effected a *cure* as much as they provided relief to the tedium of residence in hospitals. The occupations also served as a means whereby the patients might gain some benefit similar to that afforded by the idea that they were receiving help in the form of instruction in some employment, which was not only interesting at the time, but might in the future prove a means whereby they could partially be self-supporting. Work of the same kind is also still provided for the cripples and disabled men in our hospitals for paraplegias, or the St. Dunstan's Homes for the Blind. This work in such cases is found to have a distinctly beneficial effect upon the psychological health of the men, which has been influenced by their incurable condition.

It is exceedingly interesting to reflect upon the impetus given to this important subject—namely, the understanding of psycho-neuroses, as well as methods of treating them, which has been the outcome of the Great War. The appallingly large numbers who urgently required treatment because of it, made the opening of special hospitals and numerous out-patient clinics imperative to deal with the problem at the time, from which material has been collected that gives us information of results so that a comparison may be made between various methods from the point of view of cure and alleviation of cases under treatment.

Not only did it become necessary to arrange for the treatment of military patients, but also for that of civilians whose tendency to neurotic disorder had been increased through anxiety concerning relatives or their own personal safety during air-raids, among whom were men, women, and even little children. Although some of the clinics that were established had but a temporary duration, the result has been permanent; and since that time we have seen the organisation of improved departments for those suffering from nervous diseases in many of our general hospitals and separate out-patient clinics in London, as well as in the provinces, for neuroses and psycho-neuroses.

Most of the younger generation of our medical men are now aware of the impossibility to ignore the subject any longer, or to ridicule the discoveries of psycho-analysis as in the past, and feel the necessity for giving serious study to this group of human disorders. The growing interest in psycho-neuroses that is prevalent at the present day is already spreading to the nursing profession also, where it may be seen among the nursing staffs of our hospitals, our private nurses, and those engaged in school and welfare work, which is one of the most hopeful signs of the present day, since it means that thousands of our sick whose troubles have a strong bias towards neurosis will at last gain understanding, sympathy, and fair play from those upon whom they rely for real nursing, and therefore upon whom, to a very great extent, their ultimate recovery depends.

BOOKS THAT MAY BE READ IN CONNECTION WITH THIS CHAPTER

1911. *The Adolescent,* by T. W. Slaughter.

1915. *Functional Nerve Diseases and the Shock of Battle,* by David Forsyth, M.D., D.Sc., F.R.C.P.

1916. *Instincts of the Herd in Peace and War,* by W. Trotter.

1917. *War Shock. The Psychoneuroses in War,* by M. D. Eder.

1918. *Hysteria or Pithiatism,* by J. Babinski and J. Froment.

1918. *The Psychoneuroses of War,* by G. Roussey and J. L'Hermitte.

1918. *Present-day Applications of Psychology,* by Charles S. Myers, M.A., M.D., Sc.D., F.R.C.P.

1919. *Auto-erotic Phenomena in Adolescence,* by K. Menzies.

1921. *Psycho-analysis and the War Neuroses,* by Professor Dr. Sigmund Freud, Vienna; Dr. Sandor Ferenzci, Budapest; Dr. Karl Abraham, Berlin; Dr. Ernst Simmel, Berlin; Dr. Ernest Jones, London.

1926. *The Reproduction of Life,* by A. J. Cokkinis, F.R.C.S.Eng., M.B., B.S.Lond.

1928. *The Struggles of Male Adolescence,* by C. Standford Read, M.D.

BIBLIOGRAPHY

ADLER, ALFRED, DR. The Neurotic Constitution. Kegan Paul. 1918.

BABINSKI, J., and J. FROMENT. Hysteria or Pithiatism. University of London Press. 1918.

BERNFELD, DR. SIEGFRIED. The Psychology of the Infant. Kegan Paul. 1929.

BRAMWELL, J. MILNE, M.B., C.M. Hypnotism. William Rider. 1913.

BREUER, DR. JOSEF, and PROF. DR. SIGM. FREUD. Studien über Hysterie. Franz Deutike. Leipsic and Vienna. 1916.

BRIERLY, SUSAN, M.A. Introduction to Psychology. Methuen & Co. 1921.

CHADWICK, MARY. Psychology for Nurses. William Heinemann Medical Books. 1925.

Difficulties in Child Development. George Allen & Unwin. 1928.

COKKINIS, A. J., F.R.C.S.Eng., M.B., B.S.Lond. The Reproduction of Life. Baillière, Tindall & Cox. 1926.

CORIAT, DR. ISADOR. Stammering. A Psychoanalytic Interpretation. Nervous and Mental Disease Monograph Series. New York and Washington. 1928.

COUÉ, EMILE. Self-Mastery through Auto-Suggestion. George Allen & Unwin.

CRUMP, LUCY. Nursery Life 300 Years Ago. George Routledge. 1929.

CUFF, HERBERT E., M.D., F.R.C.S., and W. T. GORDON PUGH, M.D., B.C. Practical Nursing. W. Blackwood & Sons. 7th ed. 1927.

DEUTSCH, DR. HELENE. Psychoanalyse der Weiblichen Sexualfunctionen. Internationaler Psychoanalytischer Verlag. Wien. 1925.

EDER, M. D. War Shock. The Psychoneuroses in War. William Heinemann. 1917.

FORSYTH, DAVID, M.D., D.Sc., F.R.C.P. Children in Health and Disease. John Murray, 1909.

Functional Nerve Diseases and the Shock of Battle. *Lancet*, December 25, 1915, p. 1399.

Technique of Psycho-analysis. Kegan Paul. 1922.

FREUD, PROFESSOR DR. SIGMUND, LL.D. Selected papers on Hysteria and other Psychoneuroses. 1909. trans. by A. A. Brill, M.D., Ph.B. Nervous and Mental Disease Monograph Series. New York and Washington.

Totem and Taboo. George Routledge & Sons. 1919.

Psychopathology of Everyday Life. Trans. by A. A. Brill, M.D., Ph.B. Fisher Unwin.

Psycho-analysis and the War-Neuroses. Trans. published by Hogarth Press. 1921.

HART, BERNARD, M.D. Psychology of Insanity. Cambridge University Press. 1918.

HARTLEY, C. GASQUOINE. Mother and Son. Everleigh, Nash & Grayson. 1923.

JONES, ERNEST, M.D. Treatment of the Neuroses. Baillière, Tindall & Cox. 1920.

Psycho-analysis of the War-Neuroses. Trans. Hogarth Press. 1921.

JUNG, DR. C. G., LL.D. Collected Papers on Analytical Psychology. Baillière, Tindall & Cox. 1917.

Psychology of the Unconscious. Kegan Paul. 1918.

LOW, BARBARA, B.A. The Unconscious in Action. University of London Press. 1928.

MENZIES, K. Auto-Erotic Phenomena in Adolescence. H. K. Lewis, Ltd. 1919.

MYERS, CHARLES S., M.A., M.D., Sc.D., F.R.S. Present-day Applications of Psychology. Methuen & Co. 1918.

OGDEN, C. K. A B C of Psychology. Kegan Paul. 1929.

PFISTER, OSKAR. Love in Children and its Aberrations. George Allen & Unwin. 1924.

RANK, DR. OTTO. Das Trauma der Geburt. Internationaler Psychoanalytischer Verlag. Wien. 1924.

READ, C. STANDFORD, M.D. The Struggles of Male Adolescence. George Allen & Unwin. 1928.

RICKMAN, JOHN, M.D. A Survey. Development of the Psychoanalytical Theory of the Psychoses 1894–1926. Cambridge University Press. 1927.

ROUSSEY, R., and J. L'HERMITTE. The Psychoneuroses of War. University of London Press. 1918.

SACKVILLE-WEST, EDWARD. Simpson. William Heinemann. 1931.

SANDS, IRVING J., M.D. Nervous and Mental Diseases for Nurses. W. B. Saunders. 1928.

SINGER, CHARLES, M.A., M.D., D.Litt., F.R.C.P. Short History of Medicine. Oxford University Press. 1928.

SLAUGHTER, T. W. The Adolescent. George Allen & Unwin. 1911.

STEKEL, WILHELM, Dr. The Beloved Ego. Kegan Paul. 1921.

STODDART, W. H. B., M.D., F.R.C.P. Mental Nursing. The Scientific Press. 1916.

TROTTER, W. Instincts of the Herd in Peace and War. Fisher Unwin. 1916.

WHITE, WILLIAM A., M.D. Outlines of Psychiatry. Nervous and Mental Disease Monograph Series. New York & Washington. 1925.

INDEX

For Product Safety Concerns and Information please contact our EU representative GPSR@taylorandfrancis.com Taylor & Francis Verlag GmbH, Kaufingerstraße 24, 80331 München, Germany